A POCKET MANUAL OF DIFFERENTIAL DIAGNOSIS

Fourth Edition

D0285544

A POCKET MANUAL OF DIFFERENTIAL DIAGNOSIS

Fourth Edition

Stephen N. Adler, M.D., B.S.
Chief, Department of Respiratory Therapy
Mercy Health Center
Oklahoma City, Oklahoma

Dianne B. Gasbarra, M.D.
Clinical Assistant Professor of Medicine
University of Oklahoma Health Sciences Center
Private Practice
Pulmonary, Critical Care, and Internal Medicine
Mercy Health Center and Deaconess Hospital
Oklahoma City, Oklahoma

Debra Adler-Klein, M.D., F.A.C.P.
Assistant Clinical Professor of Medicine
Columbia University
College of Physicians and Surgeons
New York, New York

 LIPPINCOTT WILLIAMS & WILKINS

A **Wolters Kluwer** Company

Philadelphia · Baltimore · New York · London
Buenos Aires · Hong Kong · Sydney · Tokyo

Acquisitions Editor: Richard Winters
Developmental Editor: Erin O'Connor
Supervising Editor: Mary Ann McLaughlin
Production Editor: Shannon Garza/Silverchair Science + Communications
Manufacturing Manager: Tim Reynolds
Cover Designer: Mark Lerner
Compositor: Silverchair Science + Communications
Printer: Victor Graphics

© 2000 by LIPPINCOTT WILLIAMS & WILKINS
530 Walnut Street
Philadelphia, PA 19106-3780 USA
LWW.com

Printed in the USA

Library of Congress Cataloging-in-Publication Data

Adler, Stephen N.
  A pocket manual of differential diagnosis / Stephen N. Adler, Dianne B. Gasbarra,
  Debra Adler-Klein.-- 4th ed.
    p. cm.
  Includes bibliographical references and index.
  ISBN 0-7817-1943-7
  1. Diagnosis, Differential--Handbooks, manuals, etc. I. Gasbarra, Dianne B. II.
Adler-Klein, Debra.
  [DNLM: 1. Diagnosis, Differential--Handbooks. WB 39 A236p 1999]
RC71.5 .A341999
616.07'5 --dc21   99-042878

10 9 8 7 6 5 4 3 2

To our parents

CONTENTS

3. Drugs 61
Stephen N. Adler

4. Endocrine/Metabolic System 97
Thomas A. Murphy

5. Gastrointestinal and Hepatic Systems 151
Wendell K. Clarkston and Bruce R. Bacon

6. Genitourinary System 203
Mildred Lam

7. Hematologic System 227
Kyung-Whan Min

8. Infectious Disease 255
Debra Adler-Klein

12. Respiratory System   357
Dianne B. Gasbarra

13. Human Immunodeficiency Virus Infection 389
Debra Adler-Klein

CONTRIBUTING AUTHORS

Stephen N. Adler, M.D., B.S.
Chief, Department of Respiratory Therapy
Mercy Health Center
Oklahoma City, Oklahoma
4200 West Memorial Road
Oklahoma City, Oklahoma 73120

Debra Adler-Klein, M.D., F.A.C.P.
Assistant Clinical Professor of Medicine
Columbia University College of Physicians and Surgeons
New York, New York
Infectious Disease Associates
190 West Broad Street
Stamford, Connecticut 06902

Bruce R. Bacon, M.D.
James F. King Professor of Internal Medicine
St. Louis University School of Medicine
Director, Division of Gastroenterology
Department of Internal Medicine
St. Louis University School of Medicine
1402 South Grand Boulevard
St. Louis, Missouri 63104

Wendell K. Clarkston, M.D.
Associate Professor
Departments of Medicine, Gastroenterology, and Hepatology
University of Missouri—Kansas City School of Medicine
Kansas City, Missouri
2411 Holmes Road
Kansas City, Missouri 64108

Dianne B. Gasbarra, M.D.
Clinical Assistant Professor of Medicine
University of Oklahoma Health Sciences Center
Private Practice
Pulmonary, Critical Care, and Internal Medicine
Mercy Health Center and Deaconess Hospital
Oklahoma City, Oklahoma
4200 West Memorial Road
Suite 708
Oklahoma City, Oklahoma 73120

Mildred Lam, M.D.
Associate Professor of Medicine
Department of Medicine
Division of Nephrology
University of Virginia Health Sciences Center
Hospital West
MSB 5th Floor, Room 511
Charlottesville, Virginia 22908

Thomas A. Murphy, M.D.
Associate Professor of Medicine
Department of Medicine
Division of Endocrinology
Case Western Reserve University School of Medicine
2500 MetroHealth Drive
Cleveland, Ohio 44109

Kyung-Whan Min, M.D.
Adjunct Professor of Pathology
Univerity of Oklahoma College of Medicine
Pathologist
Deaconess Hospital
5501 N. Portland Avenue
Oklahoma City, Oklahoma 73112

PREFACE

In the practice of clinical medicine, physicians encounter a variety of symptoms, signs, and laboratory tests. Each clinical finding and test result is associated with a differential diagnosis—that is, a list of conditions or disease entities that may produce the given finding or result. Differential diagnoses for various clinical findings are available but are often scattered in a number of different references. Our book contains information gathered from many such sources, compiled in a compact, easily accessible form. It serves both as a convenient guide in the workup of clinical problems as well as a valuable teaching tool. Intended for medical students, physician's assistants, house officers, and clinicians, this book helps make the process of medical diagnosis more efficient and comprehensive. It does not, however, serve as a substitute for the thoughtful, skillful integration of data obtained by careful history-taking, physical examination, and judicious use of laboratory tests by each and every physician.

A Pocket Manual of Differential Diagnosis, Fourth Edition, has been thoroughly reviewed and updated. The continuing explosion of new pharmaceutical agents has mandated continuing changes in the text, particularly with respect to drug toxicity. Certain entries have been deleted and others expanded as the specter of human immunodeficiency virus infection continues to cast its shadow across the world. Accordingly, a new section has been devoted to this disease. The Infectious Diseases section has been completely reorganized, reflecting its importance to clinical medicine and the influence of our newest author, Dr. Debra Adler-Klein, an infectious disease clinician and teacher in Connecticut. The Eye section has been eliminated, more because of constraints of space than as a reflection of its importance to mainstream internal medicine. The new edition enjoys the entry of new writers, whom we welcome. We express thanks to all past and current contributors. Most notably, Dr. Mildred Lam, whose work has been instrumental to the quality of this book, has elected to step down to a contributing role. We acknowledge her hard work, expertise, and dedication to accuracy that contributed greatly to the success of the original and each succeeding edition.

The text is again divided into 13 chapters, ten of which are organized by organ system; the remaining three discuss acid-base and electrolyte disorders, drugs, and infectious diseases. Each chapter contains multiple entries, representing symptoms, clinical signs, laboratory tests, radiologic findings, and disease processes; approximately 200 separate entries compose the text. The differential diagnosis for each entry is listed, with more common disease entities generally being listed first. Where possible, disease entities are organized by pathophysiologic mechanism. At the end of each entry, references, usually general or subspecialty texts, are listed. Entries are cross-referenced and the book is indexed. A bibliography of general and subspecialty texts is also included at the end of each chapter.

We acknowledge the expert secretarial assistance of all who participated in the production of this manuscript, but especially that of Pat Garnett, Paul Gasbarra, and Joan Olson. Special thanks are also due to Erin O'Connor at Lippincott Williams & Wilkins for her expert help and to our editor Richard Winters, whose immediate and unconditional support made this fourth edition possible. We appreciate our families' patience and forbearance during our hours of research and manuscript preparation. Most of all, we are grateful to our many patients, who have been and shall always remain our finest teachers.

S.N.A.
D.B.G.
D.A.K.

A POCKET MANUAL OF DIFFERENTIAL DIAGNOSIS

Fourth Edition

1 ACID-BASE AND ELECTROLYTE DISORDERS

1-A. Acid-Base Nomogram

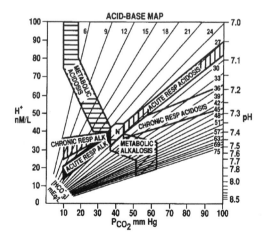

From Goldberg M, et al: Computer-Based Instruction and Diagnosis of Acid-Base Disorders. *JAMA* 1973;223:270. Copyright 1973 by the American Medical Association.

1-B. Metabolic Acidosis

Increased Anion Gap
Renal failure, acute or chronic
Ketoacidosis
    Diabetic
    Alcoholic
    Starvation
Lactic acidosis (see 1-E)
Toxins
    Aspirin
    Methanol
    Ethylene glycol
    Toluene
Nonketotic hyperosmolar coma
Inborn errors of metabolism (e.g., maple syrup urine dis-
        ease, methylmalonic aciduria)

Normal Anion Gap
Gastrointestinal loss
    Diarrhea
    Ileal loop, ureterosigmoidostomy
    Small-bowel or pancreatic fistula or drainage
    Ion-exchange resins (e.g., cholestyramine)
    Calcium or magnesium chloride ingestion
Renal loss
    Renal tubular acidosis (see 6-F)
    Hypoaldosteronism
    Carbonic anhydrase inhibitors
Recovery phase of ketoacidosis
Rapid expansion of extracellular fluid volume with bicarbonate-
        free fluid (e.g., dilutional acidosis)
Hyperalimentation with excess of cationic amino acids
Acidifying agents (e.g., ammonium chloride)

References
1. Shapiro JI, Kaehny WD: Pathogenesis and Management
   of Metabolic Acidosis and Alkalosis, p. 130. See
   Bibliography, 4.
2. Rose, p. 540. See Bibliography, 3.

1-C. Respiratory Acidosis

Neuromuscular Causes
Ingestion or overdose (e.g., tranquilizers, sedatives, anes-
        thetics, anticholinesterases)
Cerebral, brainstem, or high spinal-cord injury or infarct
Primary neuromuscular disease
    Guillain-Barré syndrome
    Myasthenia gravis
    Amyotrophic lateral sclerosis
    Poliomyelitis
    Botulism
    Tetanus
Myopathy involving respiratory muscles, especially:
    Muscular dystrophy
    Hypokalemic myopathy
    Familial periodic paralysis
Primary hypoventilation
Sleep apnea syndrome
Diaphragmatic paralysis

Airway Obstruction
Upper airway
    Laryngeal edema or spasm
    Tracheal edema, stenosis
    Obstructive sleep apnea
Lower airway
    Mechanical
        Foreign body
        Aspirated fluid (e.g., vomitus)
        Neoplasm
    Bronchospasm
        Acute
        Chronic (e.g., chronic obstructive pulmonary disease)

Cardiopulmonary-Thoracic Causes
Cardiac arrest
Severe pneumonia
Severe pulmonary edema
Respiratory distress syndrome (infant or adult)
Restrictive lung disease (e.g., interstitial fibrosis)
Massive pulmonary embolism
Pneumothorax, hemothorax
Chest trauma

Kyphoscoliosis
Smoke inhalation
Inadequate mechanical ventilation

References
1. Rose, p. 604. See Bibliography, 3.
2. Kaehny WD: Pathogenesis and Management of
   Respiratory and Mixed Acid-Base Disorders, p. 172. See
   Bibliography, 4.

1-D. Anion Gap

Increased
Without acidosis
    Administration of sodium salts of organic compounds
            (e.g., citrate, lactate, acetate)
    High-dose penicillin or carbenicillin
    Respiratory or metabolic alkalosis
    Dehydration
With acidosis
    Renal failure, acute or chronic
    Ketoacidosis
        Diabetic
        Starvation
        Alcoholic
    Nonketotic hyperosmolar coma
    Lactic acidosis (see 1-E)
    Toxins
        Aspirin
        Methanol
        Ethylene glycol
        Toluene
    Inborn errors of metabolism

Decreased
Hypoalbuminemia
Hypernatremia, severe
Dilution of extracellular fluid
Multiple myeloma
Hyperviscosity
Bromide ingestion
Hypercalcemia, hypermagnesemia (severe)
Lithium toxicity

References
1. Emmett M, Narins RG: Clinical Use of the Anion Gap. *Medicine* 56:38, 1977.
2. Rose BD, p. 545. See Bibliography, 3.

1-E. Lactic Acidosis

Associated with Impaired Tissue Oxygenation
Shock (e.g., hypovolemic, cardiogenic, septic)
Hypoxemia, respiratory failure
Anemia, severe

Occurring in Absence of Apparent Hypoxemia or Circulatory Insufficiency
Diabetes, uncontrolled
Hepatic failure
Renal failure
Malignancy, especially leukemia or lymphoma
Drugs, toxins
    Cyanide
    Carbon monoxide
    Methanol
    Salicylates
    Iron
    Strychnine
    Ethanol
Seizures
Excessive muscular activity (e.g., excessive exercise)
Alkalosis, respiratory or metabolic
D-Lactic acidosis (secondary to intestinal bacterial overgrowth)
Congenital enzyme deficiency (e.g., glycogen storage disease)

References
1. Shapiro JI, Kaehny WD: Pathogenesis and Management of Metabolic Acidosis and Alkalosis, p. 130. See Bibliography, 4.
2. Rose, p. 554. See Bibliography, 3.
3. Kreisberg RA: Lactate Homeostasis and Lactic Acidosis. *Ann Intern Med* 92:227, 1980.

1-F. Metabolic Alkalosis

Chloride-Responsive (Urine Cl⁻ <10 mEq/L)
Vomiting, nasogastric suction
Gastric drainage or fistula
Diuretics
Posthypercapnic state
Villous adenoma of colon
Congenital chloride diarrhea
Cystic fibrosis

Chloride-Resistant (Urine Cl⁻ >20 mEq/L)
Primary aldosteronism
Secondary aldosteronism
   Congestive heart failure
   Cirrhosis and ascites
   Malignant hypertension
   Adrenocorticotropic hormone (ACTH) or glucocorticoid
        excess (Cushing's disease, Cushing's syndrome,
        ectopic ACTH production)
   Bartter's syndrome
   Gitelman's syndrome
   Renin-secreting tumor (e.g., hemangiopericytoma)
Licorice ingestion
Excessive use of chewing tobacco
Severe potassium depletion
Congenital adrenal hyperplasia
Liddle's syndrome

Miscellaneous
Administration of alkali or alkalinizing agents, especially in
      the presence of renal insufficiency:
   Alkalinizing agents (e.g., citrate, lactate)
   Antacids (milk-alkali syndrome)
   Massive transfusion of blood or plasma substitute
Nonparathyroid hypercalcemia (e.g., bone metastases, multi-
      ple myeloma)
Nonreabsorbable anionic antibiotics, large doses (e.g., peni-
      cillin, carbenicillin)
Glucose ingestion after starvation

References

1. Shapiro JI, Kaehny WD: Pathogenesis and Management of Metabolic Acidosis and Alkalosis, p. 130. See Bibliography, 4.
2. Rose, p. 515. See Bibliography, 3.

1-G. Respiratory Alkalosis

Central Causes

Voluntary hyperventilation
Anxiety, pain
Hypoxia
Fever
Salicylate toxicity
Head trauma
Brain tumor
Central nervous system infection
Cerebrovascular accident
Pregnancy
Recovery phase of metabolic acidosis

Cardiopulmonary Causes

Congestive heart failure
Pneumonia
Pulmonary embolism
Interstitial lung disease
Adult respiratory distress syndrome
High altitude

Other

Hepatic insufficiency
Sepsis (especially gram-negative)
Drugs
    Progesterone, medroxyprogesterone
    Xanthines (e.g., aminophylline)
    Catecholamines (massive amounts)
    Nicotine
Mechanical ventilation
Heat exposure (e.g., heat stroke)

References

1. Rose BD, p. 629. See Bibliography, 3.
2. Kaehny WD: Pathogenesis and Management of Respiratory and Mixed Acid-Base Disorders, p. 172. See Bibliography, 4.

1-H. Hypernatremia

Pure Water Loss
Inability to obtain or swallow water (e.g., coma, dementia, infancy)
Impaired thirst drive (e.g., hypothalamic lesion)
Increased insensible loss

Excessive Sodium Intake
Iatrogenic sodium administration
  Sodium bicarbonate (cardiopulmonary resuscitation, treatment of lactic acidosis)
Accidental or deliberate ingestion of large quantities of sodium
Seawater ingestion or drowning
Mineralocorticoid or glucocorticoid excess
  Primary aldosteronism
  Cushing's syndrome
  Ectopic ACTH production

Loss of Water in Excess of Sodium (without Concomitant Water Intake)
Gastrointestinal loss (e.g., vomiting, diarrhea, intestinal fistula)
Renal loss
  Central diabetes insipidus
    Head trauma
    Posthypophysectomy
    Neoplasm
    Granulomatous disease (e.g., sarcoidosis, tuberculosis, Wegener's granulomatosis, syphilis, histiocytosis)
    Central nervous system infection
    Vascular lesion (e.g., cerebrovascular accident, aneurysm, sickle cell disease, Sheehan's syndrome)
    Congenital
  Impaired renal concentrating ability
    Osmotic diuresis
      Diabetic ketoacidosis
      Chronic renal failure, especially interstitial disease (e.g., polycystic disease, medullary cystic disease)
      Partial urinary tract obstruction, postobstructive diuresis
      Diuretic phase of acute renal failure
      Mannitol

       Tube feedings
       Infant formula (especially cow's milk)
    Excessive diuretic use
    Hypokalemia
    Hypercalcemia
    Decreased protein intake
    Prolonged, excessive water intake
    Sickle cell disease or trait
    Multiple myeloma
    Amyloidosis
    Sarcoidosis
    Sjögren's syndrome
    Nephrogenic diabetes insipidus, congenital
Drugs
    Alcohol
    Diuretics
    Lithium
    Demeclocycline
    Phenytoin
    Propoxyphene
    Sulfonylureas
    Amphotericin B
    Methoxyflurane
    Colchicine
    Vinblastine
    Foscarnet
Skin loss (e.g., burns, sweating)
Peritoneal dialysis

Essential Hypernatremia (Reset Osmostat)

References
1. Ross EJ, Christie SBM: Hypernatremia. *Medicine* 48:441, 1969.
2. Berl T, Schrier RW: Disorders of Water Metabolism, p. 1. See Bibliography, 4.

1-I. Hyponatremia

Factitious Hyponatremia (Normal Serum Osmolality)
Hyperglycemia
Hyperlipidemia

Hyperproteinemia
Hypertonic infusion of poorly reabsorbed solute (e.g., mannitol)

States with Decreased Extracellular Fluid Volume (Loss of Hypotonic Fluid Coupled with Water Intake)
Gastrointestinal loss (e.g., vomiting, diarrhea)
Third-space loss (e.g., burns, sweating, hemorrhagic pan-
        creatitis)
Renal loss
    Diuretic use
    Renal salt-wasting (e.g., advanced chronic renal failure,
        interstitial disease, renal tubular acidosis)
    Osmotic diuresis
    Mineralocorticoid deficiency

States with Increased Extracellular Fluid Volume
Congestive heart failure
Cirrhosis and ascites
Nephrotic syndrome
Renal failure, acute or chronic

States with Normal or Slightly Increased Extracellular Fluid Volume
Syndrome of inappropriate antidiuretic hormone (SIADH)
    Central nervous system disease
        Tumor
        Trauma
        Infection (meningitis, encephalitis, abscess)
        Cerebrovascular accident (thrombosis or hemorrhage)
        Guillain-Barré syndrome
        Delirium tremens
        Multiple sclerosis
    Pulmonary disease
        Tumor
        Pneumonia
        Lung abscess
        Tuberculosis
    Carcinoma (especially lung, pancreas, duodenum)
    Pain, stress (e.g., postoperative state)
    Acute psychosis
    Adrenal insufficiency
    Hypothyroidism
    Positive-pressure ventilation
    Porphyria

Drugs
   Antidiuretic hormone and analogues
   Nicotine
   Sulfonylureas (especially chlorpropamide)
   Narcotics (e.g., morphine)
   Barbiturates
   Isoproterenol
   Nonsteroidal antiinflammatory drugs
   Acetaminophen
   Clofibrate
   Carbamazepine
   Antipsychotic agents (e.g., phenothiazines)
   Antidepressants (e.g., amitriptyline, fluoxetine)
   Colchicine
   Vincristine
   Cyclophosphamide
   Ifosfamide
Psychogenic polydipsia with massive water intake (>20–25
   L/day)
Beer drinking (excessive) associated with malnutrition
Essential (reset osmostat)

References
1. Berl T, Schrier RW: Disorders of Water Metabolism, p. 1.
   See Bibliography, 4.
2. Rose, p. 651. See Bibliography, 3.

1-J. Hyperkalemia

Pseudohyperkalemia
Tourniquet use
Hemolysis (*in vitro*)
Leukocytosis, thrombocytosis

Intracellular-to-Extracellular K^+ Shift
Acidosis
Heavy exercise
Beta-blocking agents
Insulin deficiency
Digitalis intoxication
Hyperkalemic periodic paralysis
Succinylcholine

K^+ Load (Especially in Presence of Renal Insufficiency)
K^+ supplements
K^+-rich foods
K^+-containing salt substitute
Intravenous K^+
K^+-containing drugs (e.g., potassium penicillin)
Transfusion of aged blood
Hemolysis
Gastrointestinal bleeding
Cell destruction postchemotherapy (especially with leukemia,
           lymphoma, myeloma)
Rhabdomyolysis or crush injury
Extensive tissue necrosis or catabolism

Decreased K^+ Excretion
Renal failure (acute or chronic)
Drugs
     K^+-sparing diuretics (spironolactone, triamterene, amiloride)
     Beta-blocking agents
     Nonsteroidal antiinflammatory drugs
     Angiotensin converting enzyme inhibitors
     Trimethoprim
     Pentamidine
Aldosterone deficiency (see 6-F, Renal Tubular Acidosis,
           Type IV)
Selective defect in renal K^+ excretion
     Pseudohypoaldosteronism
     Lupus erythematosus
     Sickle cell disease
     Obstructive uropathy
     Renal transplantation
     Congenital

References
1. Rose, p. 823. See Bibliography, 3.
2. Peterson LN, Levi M: Disorders of Potassium Metabolism,
   p. 192. See Bibliography, 4.

1-K. Hypokalemia

Extracellular-to-intracellular K^+ shifts
     Alkalosis

Increased plasma insulin (e.g., treatment phase of dia-
 betic ketoacidosis)
Beta-adrenergic agonists
Hypokalemic periodic paralysis
Decreased intake
 Poor dietary intake
 Geophagia
Gastrointestinal loss
 Vomiting, nasogastric suction
 Diarrhea, laxative or enema abuse
 Malabsorption
 Ureterosigmoidostomy, ileal loop
 Enteric fistula
 Villous adenoma
Renal loss
 Diuretic therapy
 Primary aldosteronism
 Secondary aldosteronism
  Malignant hypertension
  Renal artery stenosis
  Congestive heart failure
  Cirrhosis and ascites
  ACTH or glucocorticoid excess (Cushing's disease,
   Cushing's syndrome, ectopic ACTH production)
  Bartter's syndrome
  Gitelman's syndrome
  Renin-secreting tumor (e.g., renal hemangiopericytoma)
 Licorice ingestion
 Excessive use of chewing tobacco
 Renal tubular acidosis
 Diuresis during recovery from obstruction or acute renal
  failure
 Osmotic diuresis
 Drugs and toxins
  Carbenicillin, penicillin (large doses)
  Amphotericin B
  L-Dopa
  Lithium
  Thallium
 Hypomagnesemia
 Acute leukemia
 Congenital adrenal hyperplasia
Sweat loss
 Heavy exercise
 Heat stroke
States of rapid cellular synthesis

Intravenous hyperalimentation
Recovery from megaloblastic anemia

References

1. Rose, p. 776. See Bibliography, 3.
2. Peterson LN, Levi M: Disorders of Potassium Metabolism, p. 192. See Bibliography, 4.

1-L. Hypercalcemia

Hemoconcentration (increased serum albumin)*
Hyperparathyroidism
    Primary
        Parathyroid adenoma
        Parathyroid hyperplasia
        Parathyroid carcinoma
        Multiple endocrine adenomatosis
    Secondary (e.g., chronic renal failure)
    Ectopic
Malignancy
    Bony metastases
    Humoral factors (e.g., parathyroid hormone–related peptide, osteoclast-activating cytokines)
    Calcium-binding globulin (multiple myeloma)*
Medications
    Thiazides
    Lithium
    Theophylline
Immobilization [in association with rapid bone turnover states (e.g., adolescence or Paget's disease)]
Milk-alkali syndrome
Vitamin D intoxication
Vitamin A intoxication
Granulomatous disease (especially sarcoidosis, tuberculosis)
Hypophosphatemia
Recovery from rhabdomyolysis-induced acute renal failure
Hyperthyroidism
Adrenal insufficiency
Acromegaly
Familial hypocalciuric hypercalcemia, other congenital causes

References
1. Popovtzer MM, Knochel JP, Kumar R: Disorders of Calcium, Phosphorus, Vitamin D, and Parathyroid Hormone Activity, p. 241. See Bibliography, 4.

*Normal serum ionized calcium.

1-M. Hypocalcemia

Hypoalbuminemia*
Vitamin D–deficiency states
    Sunlight deficiency
    Dietary deficiency
    Malabsorption (see 5-G)
        Post gastrectomy or intestinal bypass
        Sprue, tropical and nontropical
        Pancreatic insufficiency
        Hepatobiliary disease with bile salt deficiency
        Laxative abuse
    Abnormal metabolism of vitamin D
        Renal failure (acute and chronic)
        Liver failure
        Vitamin D–dependent rickets
        Anticonvulsants, microsomal enzyme inducers
Hypoparathyroidism
    Congenital
    Idiopathic (infantile- and adolescent-onset types)
    Acquired
        Surgical
        Iron overload (e.g., after multiple transfusions)
        Irradiation
        Neoplasm
Pseudohypoparathyroidism (types I and II)
Hyperphosphatemia
    Phosphate administration
        Enemas, laxatives
        Intravenous administration
        Cow's milk in infant formula
    Renal failure (chronic or acute)
    Rhabdomyolysis
    Tumor lysis syndrome

Malignancy
    Osteoblastic metastases (especially carcinoma of
          prostate, breast)
    Malignancy with increased thyrocalcitonin levels (espe-
          cially medullary carcinoma of thyroid)
Magnesium depletion (see 1-Q)
Drugs
    Loop diuretics
    Agents causing decreased bone resorption (e.g., actino-
          mycin, calcitonin, mithramycin)
    Calcium-complexing agents (e.g., citrate, ethylenedi-
          amine-tetraacetic acid)
Massive transfusion, plasma exchange
Acute pancreatitis
Healing phase of rickets, osteitis fibrosa, thyrotoxic osteopa-
          thy ("hungry bone syndrome")
Hyperkalemic periodic paralysis, acute
Osteopetrosis
Neonatal tetany

References

1. Popovtzer MM, Knochel JP, Kumar R: Disorders of
Calcium, Phosphorus, Vitamin D, and Parathyroid
Hormone Activity, p. 241. See Bibliography, 4.

*Normal serum ionized calcium.

1-N. Hyperphosphatemia

Decreased Excretion or Increased Load, or Both

Renal failure (acute or chronic)
Oral or intravenous phosphate
Phosphate-containing laxatives, enemas
Transfusion of stored blood
Acidosis (especially lactic acidosis or diabetic ketoacidosis)
Rhabdomyolysis
Tumor lysis syndrome
Hemolysis, resolving hematoma
Increased intestinal absorption (e.g., vitamin D intoxication)
Malignant hyperpyrexia
Phosphorus burns
Familial (rare)

Increased Renal Tubular Reabsorption
Hypoparathyroidism
Pseudohypoparathyroidism
Hyperthyroidism
Volume contraction
High atmospheric temperature
Postmenopausal state
Bisphosphonate therapy
Acromegaly
Juvenile hypogonadism
Tumoral calcinosis

Reference
1. Brautbar N, Kleeman CR: Hypophosphatemia and
   Hyperphosphatemia: Clinical and Pathophysiologic
   Aspects, p. 789. See Bibliography, 2.

1-O. Hypophosphatemia

Decreased Intake and Absorption and/or Increased Nonrenal Loss
Phosphate-binding antacids
Starvation, cachexia
Vomiting
Diarrhea, malabsorption
Hemodialysis

Transcellular Shift
Glucose infusion (with or without insulin administration)
Nutritional recovery syndrome
Alkalosis, respiratory
Androgens, anabolic steroids
Catecholamines (excessive secretion)
Infusion of
    Bicarbonate
    Lactate
    Glucagon
Sepsis (especially gram-negative)
Thyrotoxicosis
Heatstroke
Gout, acute
Salicylate poisoning

Pregnancy
Myocardial infarction, acute
"Hungry bone" (postparathyroidectomy) syndrome

Increased Renal Excretion
Hyperparathyroidism, primary
Diuretic therapy
Volume expansion (including hyperaldosteronism)
Hypokalemia
Hypomagnesemia
Steroid therapy, Cushing's syndrome
Estrogens, oral contraceptives
Acidosis (especially metabolic)
Renal transplantation
Renal tubular defects (e.g., Fanconi's syndrome, vitamin D–
        resistant rickets)
Tumor phosphaturia (mesenchymoma, neurofibroma, pleomor-
        phic sarcoma, sclerosing or cavernous heman-
        gioma)

Multiple Mechanisms
Alcoholism and alcoholic withdrawal
Diabetic ketoacidosis
Liver disease, hepatic coma
Hyperalimentation
Vitamin D deficiency
Recovery from severe burns

Reference
1. Popovtzer MM, Knochel JP, Kumar R: Disorders of
   Calcium, Phosphorus, Vitamin D, and Parathyroid
   Hormone Activity, p. 241. See Bibliography, 4.

1-P. Hypermagnesemia

Renal failure, acute and chronic
Increased magnesium load (especially in presence of renal
        insufficiency)
    Magnesium-containing laxatives, antacids, or enemas
    Treatment of eclampsia (mother and infant)
    Diabetic ketoacidosis
Increased renal magnesium reabsorption

Hyperparathyroidism
Familial hypocalciuric hypercalcemia
Hypothyroidism
Mineralocorticoid deficiency, adrenal insufficiency

Reference
1. Alfrey AC: Normal and Abnormal Magnesium Metabolism, p. 320. See Bibliography, 4.

1-Q. Hypomagnesemia

Redistribution
Postparathyroidectomy
Correction of metabolic acidosis (especially diabetic
             ketoacidosis)
Intravenous glucose, hyperalimentation
Refeeding after starvation
Acute pancreatitis

Decreased Intake or Increased Extrarenal Loss, or Both
Alcoholism
Malnutrition, poor intake
Nasogastric suction
Diarrhea, malabsorption (especially involving distal ileum)
Small bowel resection
Intestinal or biliary fistula
Profuse sweating, burns
Lactation

Increased Renal Loss
Drugs
    Diuretics
    Aminoglycosides
    Cisplatin
    Amphotericin B
    Cyclosporine
    Pentamidine
Alcohol abuse
Diabetic ketoacidosis
Saline or osmotic diuresis
Postobstructive or postacute renal failure diuresis
Tubulointerstitial renal disease

Hypercalcemic states
Primary or secondary aldosteronism
Potassium depletion
Hypoparathyroidism
Hyperthyroidism
SIADH
Bartter's syndrome, Gitelman's syndrome
Familial

Reference
1. Alfrey AC: Normal and Abnormal Magnesium Metabolism, p. 320. See Bibliography, 4.

Bibliography

1. Fauci AS, et al. (eds): *Harrison's Principles of Internal Medicine*, 14/e. New York: McGraw-Hill, 1998.
2. Maxwell MH, Kleeman CR, Narins RG (eds): *Clinical Disorders of Fluid and Electrolyte Metabolism*, 4/e. New York: McGraw-Hill, 1987.
3. Rose BD: *Clinical Physiology of Acid-Base and Electrolyte Disorders*, 4/e. New York: McGraw-Hill, 1994.
4. Schrier RW (ed): *Renal and Electrolyte Disorders*, 5/e. Philadelphia: Lippincott–Raven, 1997.
5. Schrier RW, Gottschalk CW (eds): *Diseases of the Kidney*, 6/e. Boston: Little, Brown and Company, 1997.

2
CARDIOVASCULAR SYSTEM

2-A. Chest Pain

Skin and subcutaneous lesions [including adiposis dolorosa,
        thrombophlebitis of thoracoepigastric vein
        (Mondor's disease)]
Breast lesions
    Fibroadenosis
    Chronic cystic mastitis
    Acute breast abscess or mastitis
    Carcinoma
Musculoskeletal disorders
    Bruised or fractured rib
    Periostitis
    Periosteal hematoma
    Costochondritis (Tietze's syndrome)
    Slipping costal cartilage
    Intercostal muscle "stitch" or cramp
    Intercostal myositis
    Pectoral or other muscular strain
    Shoulder girdle disorders (e.g., subacromial bursitis)
    Cervical disc herniation
    Dorsal spine osteoarthritis
    Thoracic outlet syndrome
Neuralgia
    Herpes zoster
    Tabes dorsalis
    Neurofibroma
    Neoplasm

Pericardial disease
  Pericarditis (see 2-I)
  Neoplasm
  Congenital absence of left pericardium
Mediastinal disease
  Mediastinal emphysema
  Neoplasm
  Mediastinitis
Cardiovascular disease
  Acute myocardial infarction
  Angina pectoris
  Aortic valvular disease
  Hypertrophic cardiomyopathy
  Mitral valve prolapse
  Acute aortic dissection
  Thoracic aortic aneurysm
  Myocarditis
  Primary pulmonary hypertension
  Ruptured sinus of Valsalva aneurysm
Pleural or pulmonary disease
  Pleuritis of any etiology (e.g., pneumothorax; see 12-F)
  Tracheobronchitis
  Pneumonia
  Pulmonary hypertension (see 12-O)
  Pulmonary thromboembolism
  Neoplasm
    Bronchogenic carcinoma
    Metastatic tumor
    Mesothelioma
    Other parenchymal lesions
Gastrointestinal disease
  Esophageal lesions
    Esophagitis
    Esophageal spasm
    Mallory-Weiss syndrome
    Esophageal rupture
    Foreign body
    Carcinoma
    Zenker's diverticulum
    Plummer-Vinson syndrome
  Peptic ulcer disease (with or without perforation)
  Gastric distention
  Gastritis
    Biliary disease
    Acute cholecystitis
    Biliary colic
  Distention of the liver

Pancreatitis
Subphrenic abscess
Splenic infarct
Splenic flexure syndrome
Thyroiditis
Psychogenic causes

References
1. Williams, ES: Approach to the Patient with Chest Pain, p. 317. See Bibliography, 5.
2. Braunwald E: The History, p. 1. See Bibliography, 1.

2-B. Edema

Localized
Venous or lymphatic obstruction and/or insufficiency
Venous thrombosis
Baker's cyst
Tumor invasion or compression (e.g., superior vena cava syndrome)
Surgical or radiation damage
Filariasis
Inflammatory disease
Allergic process
Physical or chemical trauma
Stings and bites
Immobilized or paralyzed limb
Congenital lymphedema

Generalized
Biventricular congestive heart failure (see 2-G)
Tricuspid stenosis
Cor pulmonale (see 12-O)
Pericardial disease (see 2-I, 2-J)
Chronic constrictive pericarditis
Pericardial effusion
Hypoalbuminemic states
Hepatic cirrhosis
Nephrotic syndrome
Protein-losing enteropathy
Malnutrition
Severe chronic disease
Acute and chronic renal failure with volume overload

Inferior vena cava obstruction
Myxedema
Pregnancy
Iatrogenic salt overload
    Enteral feeding
    Intravenous fluid administration
    Drugs
        Carbenicillin and similar drugs
        Tamoxifen
        Estrogens
        Corticosteroids
        Minoxidil
        Calcium channel blockers (e.g., nifedipine)
        Guanethidine
        Diazoxide
Trichinosis
Idiopathic cyclic edema
Hereditary angioneurotic edema

References

1. Perloff JK, Braunwald E: Physical Examination of the Heart and Circulation, p. 15. See Bibliography, 1.
2. Shayman JA: Approach to the Patient with Edema, p. 948. See Bibliography, 3.

2-C. Palpitation*

Palpitation without Arrhythmia
Noncardiac disorders
    Anxiety
    Exercise
    Anemia
    Fever
    Volume depletion
    Postural hypotension
    Thyrotoxicosis
    Menopausal syndrome
    Hypoglycemia
    Pheochromocytoma
    Aortic aneurysm
    Migraine syndrome
    Arteriovenous fistula
    Diaphragmatic flutter

Drugs
    Sympathomimetic agents
    Ganglionic blockers
    Digitalis
    Nitrates
    Aminophylline
    Atropine
    Coffee, tea
    Tobacco
    Alcohol
    Thyroid extract
Cardiac disorders
    Aortic regurgitation
    Aortic stenosis
    Patent ductus arteriosus
    Ventricular septal defect
    Atrial septal defect
    Marked cardiomegaly
    Acute left ventricular failure
    Hyperkinetic heart syndrome
    Tricuspid insufficiency
    Pericarditis
    Prosthetic heart valve
    Electronic pacemaker

Palpitation with Arrhythmia (see 2-O)

Extrasystoles
Bradyarrhythmias
Tachyarrhythmias

Reference

1. Goldman L: Chest Discomfort and Palpitation, p. 58. See Bibliography, 2.

*Palpitation is the sensation of disturbed heartbeat. This entry was modified from Shander D: Palpitation and Disorders of Heartbeat, p. 117. See Bibliography, 2.

2-D. Hypertension*

Systolic and Diastolic

Pseudohypertension (e.g., wrong-sized cuff)

Primary (essential)
Renal causes
    Parenchymal
    Vascular
    Renoprival (after bilateral nephrectomy)
    Renin-producing tumor
    Liddle's syndrome
Endocrine causes
    Acromegaly
    Hypothyroidism
    Hypercalcemia
    Adrenal causes
        Congenital adrenal hyperplasia
        Cushing's syndrome
        Primary aldosteronism
        Pheochromocytoma
    Extraadrenal chromaffin tumors
    Exogenous
        Oral contraceptives
        Estrogens
        Glucocorticoids
        Mineralocorticoids (e.g., licorice)
        Sympathomimetic agents
        Tyramine-containing foods and monoamine oxidase
            inhibitors
Coarctation of aorta
Pregnancy-induced
Neurogenic causes
    Increased intracranial pressure
    Postoperative state
    Acute porphyria
    Lead poisoning
    Quadriplegia (acute)
    Diencephalic syndrome
    Familial dysautonomia
Increased intravascular volume
    Polycythemia vera
    Iatrogenic causes
Burns
Sleep apnea
Psychogenic causes
Drug withdrawal
Other drugs
    Cocaine
    Cyclosporine
    Erythropoietin

Systolic
Increased cardiac output or stroke volume, or both
    Aortic valvular regurgitation
    Fever
    Arteriovenous fistula, patent ductus arteriosus
    Paget's disease
    Beriberi
    Thyrotoxicosis (endogenous or exogenous)
    Anemia
    Hyperkinetic circulation
    Anxiety
    Complete heart block
Aortic rigidity

References
1. Kaplan NM: Systemic Hypertension: Mechanisms and Diagnosis, p. 807. See Bibliography, 1.
2. Weinberger, MH: Systemic Hypertension, p. 175. See Bibliography, 5.

*Modified from Kaplan NM: Systemic Hypertension: Mechanisms and Diagnosis, p. 811. See Bibliography, 1.

2-E. Jugular Venous Distention

Extrathoracic Causes
Local venous obstruction of any cause (e.g., cervical goiter)
Circulatory overload of noncardiac etiology

Intrathoracic Causes
Valsalva maneuver
Retrosternal goiter
Superior vena cava syndrome
    Benign
    Malignant
Pericardial disease (see 2-I, 2-J)
    Cardiac tamponade
    Constrictive pericarditis
Cardiac disease
    Right or left heart failure, or both, of any etiology (e.g., tricuspid valve disease; see 2-G)

Restrictive cardiomyopathy
Right atrial myxoma
Hyperkinetic heart circulatory states
Pleuropulmonary disease
Pulmonary hypertension of any etiology (see 12-O)
Bronchial asthma
Chronic bronchitis and emphysema
Tension pneumothorax

Reference

1. Friedman HH: Jugular Venous Pulse, p. 49. See Bibliography, 4.

2-F. Heart Murmurs*

Systolic
Early systolic
Physiologic (innocent)
Small ventricular septal defect
Large ventricular septal defect with pulmonary hypertension
Severe acute mitral or tricuspid regurgitation
Tricuspid regurgitation without pulmonary hypertension
Midsystolic
Physiologic (innocent)
Vibratory murmur
Hyperkinetic states
Pulmonary ejection murmur
Aortic ejection murmur of old age
Obstruction to left ventricular outflow
Valvular aortic stenosis
Supravalvular aortic stenosis
Hypertrophic cardiomyopathy
Aortic valve prosthesis
Aortic dilatation
Murmurs of mitral regurgitation (occasionally)
Aortic flow murmur in aortic regurgitation
Coarctation of aorta
Supraclavicular arterial bruit
Obstruction to right ventricular outflow
Supravalvular pulmonary arterial stenosis
Pulmonic valvular stenosis
Subpulmonic (infundibular) stenosis
Flow murmur of atrial septal defect

Idiopathic dilatation of pulmonary artery
Pulmonary hypertension of any cause (occasionally)
Late systolic
Mitral valve prolapse
Tricuspid valve prolapse
Holosystolic
Mitral regurgitation
Tricuspid regurgitation secondary to pulmonary hyperten-
sion
Ventricular septal defect
Patent ductus arteriosus or aorticopulmonary window with
pulmonary hypertension

Diastolic
Early diastolic
Aortic regurgitation
Pulmonic regurgitation associated with pulmonary hyper-
tension, congenital or valvular disease
Middiastolic
Mitral stenosis
Mitral valve prosthesis
Tricuspid stenosis
Atrial myxoma
Left atrial ball-valve thrombus
Austin Flint murmur
Increased diastolic atrioventricular flow
Hyperkinetic states
Mitral and tricuspid regurgitation
Left-to-right shunt (e.g., ventricular septal defect)
Acute rheumatic valvulitis
Complete heart block
Coronary artery stenosis
Presystolic
Mitral stenosis
Tricuspid stenosis
Atrial myxoma
Left-to-right shunt
Complete heart block
Severe pulmonic stenosis
Fourth heart sound
Severe aortic insufficiency

Continuous
Pseudomurmur (e.g., pericardial friction rub)
Traumatic or surgical arteriovenous fistula

Patent ductus arteriosus
Surgically created aorticopulmonary fistula
Pulmonary arteriovenous fistula
Aorticopulmonary window without severe pulmonary
          hypertension
Pulmonary embolism
Coronary arteriovenous fistula
Ruptured sinus of Valsalva aneurysm
Coarctation of aorta
Bronchial artery collateral circulation
Lutembacher's syndrome
Anomalous left coronary artery
Intercostal arteriovenous fistula
Cervical venous hum
Mammary souffle
Aortic arch syndrome
Pulmonary artery branch stenosis or partial occlusion

References

1. Craige E, Braunwald E: The Physical Examination, p. 35.
   See Bibliography, 1.
2. Williams ES: Essential Features of the Cardiac History
   and Physical Examination, p. 315. See Bibliography, 2.
3. Friedman HH: Cardiovascular Problems: Heart Murmurs,
   p. 74. See Bibliography, 4.

*See also 2-N.

2-G. Congestive Heart Failure

Left Heart Failure
Hypertensive heart disease
Coronary artery disease
Left ventricular diastolic dysfunction
Acute myocardial infarction
Aortic and mitral valvular disease
Cardiomyopathy (see 2-H)
Pericardial disease (see 2-I, 2-J)
Arrhythmias
Congenital heart disease
Endocarditis
Cardiotoxic drugs (e.g., Adriamycin)
Myocarditis

Acute rheumatic fever
Traumatic heart disease
Thyrotoxicosis
Thiamine deficiency
Anemia
Arteriovenous fistula (e.g., Paget's disease)
Neoplastic heart disease
Toxic shock syndrome
Pulmonary thromboembolism
Postcardioversion
Pregnancy
Left atrial thrombus

Right Heart Failure*

Associated with pulmonary venous hypertension (postcapillary)
    Cardiac disease (see previous Left Heart Failure)
    Pulmonary venous disease
        Mediastinal neoplasm or granuloma
        Mediastinitis and fibrosis
        Anomalous pulmonary venous return
        Congenital pulmonary venous stenosis
        Idiopathic pulmonary veno-occlusive disease
Associated with pulmonary arterial hypertension (precapillary)
    Lung and pleural disease
        Chronic bronchitis, emphysema, and asthma
        Granulomatous disease (e.g., sarcoidosis)
        Pneumonia
        Fibrotic disease
        Neoplasm
        Chronic suppurative disease (e.g., bronchiectasis)
        Cystic fibrosis
        Collagen-vascular disease
        Other restrictive processes (see 12-N)
        After lung resection
        Bronchopulmonary dysplasia
        Fibrothorax
    Chest wall deformity
        Kyphoscoliosis
        Thoracoplasty
    Congenital pulmonary hypoplasia (Down syndrome)
    Alveolar hypoventilation
        Neuromuscular
        Primary alveolar hypoventilation
        Obesity
        Sleep apnea syndrome
    High-altitude pulmonary hypertension

Intracardiac disease
  Increased flow associated with large left-to-right shunt
    Patent ductus arteriosus
    Atrial septal defect
    Ventricular septal defect
    Sinus of Valsalva aneurysm
  Decreased flow
    Tetralogy of Fallot
    Peripheral pulmonary artery stenosis (or stenoses)
    Unilateral absence or stenosis of pulmonary artery
Vascular disease (see 12-O)
  Pulmonary thromboembolic disease
  Primary pulmonary hypertension
  Hepatic cirrhosis and/or partial thrombosis
  Chemically induced (e.g., aminorex)
  Persistent fetal circulation
  Pulmonary arteritis
  Peripheral pulmonary artery stenosis
  Unilateral stenosis or absence of pulmonary artery
Without pulmonary hypertension
  Pulmonic stenosis
  Tricuspid stenosis (nonrheumatic)
  Tricuspid regurgitation not associated with pulmonary
      hypertension
  Decreased right ventricular compliance
  Ebstein's anomaly
  Atrial myxoma

Reference
1. Grossman W, Braunwald E: Pulmonary Hypertension, p. 780. See Bibliography, 1.

*See 12-O.

2-H. Cardiomyopathy*

Dilated
Congenital
  Familial
  Duchenne's muscular dystrophy
  Facioscapulohumeral muscular dystrophy
  Limb-girdle muscular dystrophy
  Myotonic dystrophy
  Refsum disease

    Friedreich's ataxia
Acquired
    Idiopathic
    Inflammatory
        Infective myocarditis (eg. Chagas' disease,
            Coxsackie virus)
        Acquired immunodeficiency syndrome
        Noninfective
            Collagen diseases
            Giant cell myocarditis
            Kawasaki disease
Metabolic
    Hypoxia
    Nutritional
        Thiamine deficiency
        Kwashiorkor
        Pellagra
        Scurvy
        Hypervitaminosis D
        Obesity
        Selenium deficiency
        Carnitine deficiency
    Endocrine
        Acromegaly
        Thyrotoxicosis
        Myxedema
        Uremia
        Cushing's disease
        Pheochromocytoma
        Diabetes
        Hypophosphatemia
        Hypocalcemia
    Altered metabolism
        Gout
        Porphyria
        Oxalosis
    Electrolyte imbalance
Toxins, drugs
    Alcohol
    Disopyramide
    Daunorubicin
    Doxorubicin (Adriamycin)
    Cyclophosphamide
    Cocaine
    Bleomycin
    5-Fluorouracil
    Phosphate (poisoning)

    Phenothiazines and antidepressants
    Lithium
    Carbon monoxide
    Emetine
    Chloroquine
    Acetaminophen, paracetamol
    Lead
    Arsenic
    Hydrocarbons
    Antimony
    Cobalt
    Snake or insect bites
Infiltrative
    Right ventricular dysplasia
    Collagen vascular disease
    Amyloidosis
    Hemochromatosis
    Neoplastic
    Sarcoidosis
    Whipple's disease
Hematologic
    Leukemia
    Thrombotic thrombocytopenic purpura
    Sickle cell anemia
    Polycythemia vera
Hypersensitivity
    Methyldopa
    Penicillin
    Sulfonamides
    Tetracycline
    Phenindione
    Giant cell myocarditis
    Cardiac transplant rejection
Peripartum
Vasculitis
Physical agents
    Irradiation
    Trauma
    Heatstroke
    Hypothermia
    Chronic tachycardia

Restrictive
Pseudocardiomyopathy (i.e., constrictive pericarditis)
Amyloidosis
Idiopathic (familial and nonfamilial)

Hemochromatosis
Sarcoidosis
Scleroderma
Diabetic
Pseudoxanthoma elasticum
Neoplasm
Endocardial fibroelastosis
Fatty infiltration
Drugs
   Serotonin
   Ergotamine
   Busulfan
   Methysergide
   Mercurials
Löffler's endocarditis (hypereosinophilic syndrome)
Endomyocardial fibrosis
Carcinoid heart disease
Whipple's disease
Fabry's disease
Glycogen storage disease
Gaucher's disease
Hurler's disease
Sphingolipidosis

Hypertrophic
Idiopathic hypertrophic cardiomyopathy
Idiopathic nonobstructive cardiomyopathy
Glycogen storage disease (Pompe's disease)
Friedreich's ataxia
Lentiginosis

References
1. Wynne J, Braunwald E: The Cardiomyopathies and Myocarditides, p. 1404. See Bibliography, 1.
2. Dec GW, Fuster V: Idiopathic Dilated Cardiomyopathy. *N Engl J Med* 331:1564–1575, 1994.
3. Kushwaha SS, Fallon JT, Fuster V: Restrictive Cardiomyopathy. *N Engl J Med* 336:267–276, 1997.

*The distinction between cardiomyopathy by functional impairment is not absolute and overlap occurs frequently.

2-I Pericarditis*

Idiopathic[†]
Infection
    Viral [e.g., acquired immunodeficiency syndrome (AIDS)][†]
    Bacterial[†]
    Mycobacterial[†]
    Mycoplasmal
    Fungal[†]
    Parasitic[†]
    Spirochetal (e.g., Lyme disease)
Acute myocardial infarction
Uremia[†]
Neoplasm[†]
Aortic dissection with hemopericardium
Connective-tissue or hypersensitivity diseases[†]
    Postmyocardial infarction (Dressler's syndrome)
    Postpericardiotomy
    Drugs
        Penicillin
        Methysergide
        Daunorubicin and doxorubicin
        Minoxidil
        Dantrolene
        Bleomycin
        Cyclophosphamide
        Practolol
    Systemic lupus erythematosus
        Idiopathic
        Drug-related
            Hydralazine
            Procainamide
            Phenytoin
            Isoniazid
            Methyldopa
    Mixed connective-tissue disease
    Scleroderma
    Wegener's granulomatosis
    Rheumatoid arthritis
    Polyarteritis nodosa
    Polymyositis
    Reiter's syndrome
    Ankylosing spondylitis
    Serum sickness

Acute rheumatic fever
Trauma[†]
    Penetrating wounds
    Catheter- or pacemaker-induced cardiac
          perforation
    Blunt chest trauma
    Cardiopulmonary resuscitation
    Cardiothoracic surgery
    Cardioversion
    Pancreatic-pericardial fistula
Chylopericardium
Pseudoaneurysm neptune
Cholesterol pericarditis
    Idiopathic
    Rheumatoid arthritis
    Hypercholesterolemia
    Myxedema
    Tuberculosis
Talc or other foreign substance
Sarcoidosis
Postirradiation[†]
Esophageal rupture
Uncommon miscellaneous etiologies
    Congenital heart disease (e.g., atrial septal defect)
    Familial Mediterranean fever
    Right atrial myxoma
    Degos' disease
    Gaucher's disease
    Myeloid metaplasia
    Amyloidosis
    Silicosis
    Giant cell arteritis
    Scorpion fish sting
    Pseudomyxoma peritonei
    Severe chronic anemia (e.g., thalassemia)
    Pancreatitis
    Whipple's disease
    Acute gouty arthritis
    Associated with atrial septal defect
    Pulmonary thromboembolism
    Takayasu's disease
    Mulibrey nanism[†]
    Nontraumatic hemopericardium
    Inflammatory bowel disease
    Behçet's disease

References

1. Lorell BH, Braunwald E: Pericardial Disease, p. 1478. See Bibliography, 1.
2. Hancock IW: Pericardial Diseases, p. 461. See Bibliography, 5.

---

*See also 2-J.
†May be commonly associated with development of constrictive pericarditis.

2-J. Pericardial Effusion

Pericarditis of any cause* (see 2-I)
Congestive heart failure
Hypoalbuminemia
Cirrhosis
Nephrotic syndrome
Malnutrition
Chronic disease
Acute pancreatitis
Chylopericardium*
    Congenital, idiopathic
    Neoplasm (e.g., lymphoma)
    After cardiothoracic surgery
    Benign obstruction of thoracic duct
Hemopericardium†
    Trauma
        Blunt and/or penetrating
        Iatrogenic
    Anticoagulants
    Chemotherapeutic agents
    Myocardial infarction
    Cardiac rupture
    Aortic or pulmonary artery rupture
    Coagulopathy
    Uremia
Myxedema*

References

1. Lorell BH, Braunwald E: Pericardial Disease, p. 1485. See Bibliography, 1.

2. Roberts WC, Spray TL: Pericardial Heart Disease. *Curr Prob Cardiol* 2(3):55, 1977.

*May be associated with chronic constrictive pericarditis.
†May be associated with acute cardiac tamponade.

2-K. Hypotension and Shock

Hypovolemia
    External losses
        Hemorrhage
        Gastrointestinal loss
        Fistulae
        Renal loss
            Diuretics
            Diabetes insipidus
            Osmotic diuresis (e.g., diabetes mellitus)
            Diuretic phase of acute renal failure
            Salt-losing nephropathy
            Postobstructive diuresis
        Cutaneous loss
            Burns
            Exudative lesions
            Perspiration and insensible loss without replacement
    Internal losses
        Hemorrhage (e.g., anticoagulant therapy)
            Hemothorax
            Hemoperitoneum
            Retroperitoneal hemorrhage
            Soft tissue injury
            Fracture
        Fluid sequestration
            Ascites
            Bowel obstruction or infarction
            Peritonitis
            Phlegmon (e.g., pancreatitis)
            Budd-Chiari syndrome
Cardiovascular causes
    Arrhythmia (see 2-O)
    Regurgitant lesions
        Acute mitral or aortic regurgitation
        Rupture of interventricular septum
        Giant left ventricular aneurysm

Obstructive lesions
    Valvular stenosis
    Hypertrophic cardiomyopathy
    Atrial myxoma
    Intracardiac or valvular thrombus (including prosthetic
        valve)
Myopathy
    Acute myocardial infarction
    Contusion
    Dilated or restrictive cardiomyopathy (see 2-H)
    Ventricular wall defects and aneurysms
    Other myocardial disorders (associated with low car-
        diac output) (see 2-G)
Pericardial disease (see 2-I, 2-J)
    Cardiac tamponade
    Constrictive pericarditis
Aortic lesions
    Acute dissection
    Coarctation
    Rupture (e.g., trauma or aneurysm)
Congenital heart disease
Vena cava obstruction
Pleuropulmonary disease
    Tension pneumothorax
    Positive pressure ventilation
    Pulmonary embolism (including thrombus, amniotic fluid,
        air, tumor)
    Primary or secondary pulmonary hypertension
    Eisenmenger reaction
Infection
    Septicemia
    Specific infections (e.g., dengue fever)
    Toxic shock syndrome
Anaphylaxis
Endocrine disease
    Adrenal insufficiency
    Hypoglycemia or hyperglycemia
    Hypocalcemia or hypercalcemia
    Myxedema or thyroid storm
    Pheochromocytoma
    Pituitary failure including diabetes insipidus
Hypoxia
Severe acidosis or alkalosis
Nonbacterial sepsis syndrome
Hypothermia or hyperthermia
Hepatic failure

Drugs and toxins
    Drug overdose and poisoning (e.g., barbiturates)
    Antihypertensive agents
    Other vasodilators (e.g., nitroglycerin)
    Heavy metals
    Anesthesia (e.g., propofol)
    Polycythemia vera
    Sickle cell crisis
Hyperviscosity syndrome
Neuropathic causes
    Brainstem failure
    Spinal cord dysfunction
    Autonomic insufficiency

References

1. Leier CV: Approach to the Patient with Hypotension and Shock, p. 361. See Bibliography, 5.
2. Jimenez EJ: Shock, p. 359. See Bibliography, 5.

2-L. Cardiac Arrest (Sudden Cardiopulmonary Collapse)

Arrhythmia (with or without digitalis intoxication)
    Tachyarrhythmia
        Ventricular fibrillation (e.g., prolonged QT syndromes)
        Ventricular tachycardia
    Bradyarrhythmia
        Sinus bradycardia
        Junctional rhythm
        Atrioventricular block
        Idioventricular rhythm
    Asystole
Upper airway obstruction
    Structural lesion
    Sleep apnea syndrome
    Foreign body
Acute and/or chronic respiratory failure with hypoxemia and/or hypercarbia (see 12-M)
Hypoxia of any cause (e.g., carbon monoxide poisoning)
Pulmonary hypertension
Smoke inhalation
Severe acidosis or alkalosis

Hypoglycemia
Syncope (see 11-D)
Addisonian crisis
Drug overdose, allergy, or adverse reaction
   Narcotics
   Insulin
   Sedatives
   Digitalis
   Quinidine
   Cocaine
   Disopyramide
   Procainamide and other antiarrhythmics
   Phenothiazines
   Tricyclic antidepressants
   Nitrates
   Aminophylline
   Propranolol
   Warfarin
   Penicillins
   Sulfonamides
   Antihypertensive agents
Shock of any etiology (see also 2-K), especially
   Hypovolemia
   Tension pneumothorax
   Cardiac tamponade or pericardial constriction
   Anaphylaxis
   Sepsis
   Aortic dissection or rupture
   Pulmonary embolism (of any type)
   Acute myocardial infarction
   Other common cardiac causes
      Severe coronary heart disease
      Hypertensive heart disease
      Valvular disease (e.g., aortic stenosis; see 2-N)
      Prosthetic valve dysfunction or thrombosis
      Myocarditis and cardiomyopathy (see 2-H)
      Cardiac rupture
      Congenital heart disease including anomalous coro-
         nary artery anatomy
      Mitral valve prolapse
      Primary conduction system or nodal disease
      Intracardiac thrombosis
      Nonatherosclerotic obstruction of coronary arteries
         Embolus
         Arteritis
         Dissection (e.g., in pregnancy, Marfan's)

Spasm
Congenital anomalies
Coronary artery ostia obstruction (e.g., syphilis)
Electrolyte abnormality (especially potassium, calcium, magnesium)
Hypothermia or hyperthermia
Electric shock
Drowning
Insect stings and bites
Neurologic disorders
Stroke
Hemorrhage
Seizure
Brainstem compression of any cause
Infection
Sudden infant death syndrome
Liquid protein diet
Modified fast diet programs

References

1. Myerburg RJ, Castellanos A: Cardiovascular Arrest and Sudden Cardiac Death, p. 742. See Bibliography, 1.
2. Myerburg RJ, Castellanos A: Cardiovascular Collapse, Cardiac Arrest and Sudden Cardiac Disease, p. 221. See Bibliography, 2.

2-M. Complications of Cardiopulmonary Resuscitation

Cerebral
Hypoxic encephalopathy
Oronasopharyngeal
Laceration
Fractured teeth
Epistaxis
Laryngeal injury
Neck
Spinal cord injury
Vascular injury and hematoma
Lung and chest wall
Pneumothorax and pneumomediastinum
Subcutaneous emphysema

Rib and sternal fractures
Hemothorax
Pulmonary contusion
Atelectasis
    Malpositioned endotracheal tube
    Foreign body
    Secretions
Aspiration
Heart and pericardium
    Hemopericardium and cardiac tamponade
    Lacerated heart or coronary vessels
    Ruptured ventricle
Visceral injury
    Acute gastric dilatation
    Gastroesophageal, liver, or splenic laceration
Acute renal failure
Fat embolism
Volume overload
Metabolic alkalosis
    Sodium bicarbonate administration
    Posthypercapnic
Bacteremia

Reference

1. Myerburg RJ, Castellanos A: Cardiovascular Arrest and Sudden Cardiac Death, p. 742. See Bibliography, 1.

2-N. Valvular Disease*

Aortic Valve
Stenosis
    Valvular
        Congenital
        Rheumatic
        Calcific (senile)
        Atherosclerotic
        Rheumatoid
        Ochronosis
    Supravalvular
    Subvalvular
Regurgitation
    Congenital
        Bicuspid aortic valve

Isolated
Associated with
 Coarctation
 Ventricular septal defect
 Patent ductus arteriosus
Tricuspid aortic valve
 Isolated
 Associated with
  Ventricular septal defect
  Valvular aortic stenosis
  Supravalvular aortic stenosis
  Subvalvular aortic stenosis
  Congenital aneurysm of sinus of Valsalva
  Cusp fenestrations
Quadricuspid aortic valve
Acquired
 Valvular
  Rheumatic heart disease
  Bacterial endocarditis
  Calcific aortic valve disease
  Atherosclerosis
  Traumatic valve rupture
  Dissection of the aorta
  Post–aortic valve surgery
   Postvalvulotomy
   Leakage around prosthesis
   Endocarditis
  Miscellaneous
   Ankylosing spondylitis
   Reiter's syndrome
   Rheumatoid arthritis
   Whipple's disease
   Crohn's disease
   Jaccoud's arthropathy
   Systemic lupus erythematosus
   Scleroderma
   Myxomatous degeneration
   Pseudoxanthoma elasticum
   Mucopolysaccharidoses
   Osteogenesis imperfecta
   Cusp fenestrations
   Methysergide
 Aortic dilatation or distortion
  Senile dilatation
  Cystic medial necrosis with or without Marfan's
   syndrome

Takayasu's disease
Relapsing polychondritis
Syphilis
Ankylosing spondylitis
Psoriatic arthritis
Ulcerative colitis with arthritis
Reiter's syndrome
Giant cell arteritis
Ehlers-Danlos syndrome
Hypertension
Cogan's syndrome
Behçet's syndrome

Mitral Valve
Stenosis
  Congenital
  Rheumatic
  Carcinoid syndrome
  Marantic endocarditis
  Systemic lupus erythematosus
  Calcific
  Lutembacher's syndrome
  Amyloidosis
  Rheumatoid arthritis
  Hunter-Hurler disease
  Methysergide
Regurgitation
  Congenital
    Isolated mitral regurgitation
    Hypertrophic cardiomyopathy
    Connective tissue disorders
      Ehlers-Danlos syndrome
      Hurler's syndrome
      Marfan's syndrome
      Pseudoxanthoma elasticum
      Osteogenesis imperfecta
    Atrioventricular cushion defect
    Endocardial fibroelastosis
    Parachute mitral valve complex
    Hypoplastic left heart syndrome
    Anomalous left coronary artery from pulmonary artery
    Congenital mitral stenosis
    Corrected transposition of great vessels with or without
        Ebstein's malformation
    Supravalvular ring of left atrium

Acquired
  Coronary heart disease
  Rheumatic (acute or chronic)
  Mitral valve prolapse syndrome
  Papillary muscle dysfunction
    Coronary heart disease with or without myocardial
        infarction
    Neoplasm
    Myocardial abscess
    Granulomas
    Sarcoidosis
    Amyloidosis
  Ruptured or abnormal chordae tendineae (e.g., idio-
      pathic myxomatous proliferation)
  Bacterial endocarditis
  Calcified mitral annulus
    Idiopathic systemic hypertension
    Aortic stenosis
    Diabetes
    Chronic renal failure with secondary hyperparathy-
        roidism
  Left ventricular dilatation or aneurysm (e.g., dilated
      cardiomyopathy)
  Aortic valve disease
  Prosthetic valve disruption
  Trauma
  Post–cardiac surgery
  Rheumatoid arthritis
  Ankylosing spondylitis
  Scleroderma
  Systemic lupus erythematosus
  Left atrial myxoma
  Spontaneous rupture
  Carcinoid syndrome
  Giant left atrium
  Kawasaki disease
  Hypereosinophilic syndrome

Pulmonic Valve
Stenosis
  Congenital
    Valvular stenosis
    Valvular dysplasia (e.g., Noonan's syndrome)
    Tetralogy of Fallot
    Supravalvular aortic stenosis syndrome

Acquired
    Intrinsic valvular lesions
        Rheumatic disease
        Carcinoid syndrome
        Endocarditis
        Primary neoplasm
    Extrinsic lesions
        Neoplasm
        Aortic or septal aneurysm
        Sinus of Valsalva aneurysm
        Constrictive pericarditis
Regurgitation
    Congenital
        Absent pulmonic valve
        Isolated pulmonic regurgitation
        Associated with:
            Tetralogy of Fallot
            Ventricular septal defect
            Pulmonic valvular stenosis
            Idiopathic dilatation of pulmonic valve
    Acquired
        Valve ring dilatation secondary to pulmonary hypertension of any cause (see 2-G, Right Heart Failure)
        Pulmonary artery dilatation, idiopathic
        Bacterial endocarditis
        Post–pulmonic valve surgery
        Rheumatic disease
        Trauma
        Syphilis
        Carcinoid syndrome
        Marfan's syndrome
        Induced by pulmonary artery catheter

Tricuspid Valve

Stenosis
    Rheumatic heart disease (acute and chronic)
    Carcinoid syndrome
    Fibroelastosis
    Tricuspid atresia
    Endomyocardial fibrosis
Regurgitation
    Right ventricular dilatation of any cause (e.g., mitral stenosis)
    Pulmonary hypertension (see 2-G, Right Heart Failure)
    Rheumatic heart disease
    Right ventricular papillary muscle dysfunction

Myxomatous valve and chordae (usually in association
with mitral valve prolapse with or without atrial
septal defect)
Trauma
Bacterial endocarditis
Carcinoid syndrome
Ebstein's anomaly
Common atrioventricular canal
Ventricular septal aneurysm
Right atrial myxoma
Constrictive pericarditis
Endomyocardial fibrosis
Methysergide
Systemic lupus erythematosus
Radiation injury
Thyrotoxicosis
Isolated lesion
After surgical excision
Marfan's syndrome
Rheumatoid arthritis

References
1. Braunwald E: Valvular Heart Disease, p. 1007. See
   Bibliography, 1.
2. Weiss JL: Valvular Heart Disease, p. 435. See
   Bibliography, 5.

*See also 2-F.

2-O. Arrhythmias

Premature Beats
Extrasystole
   Sinus (rare)
   Atrial
   Atrioventricular junctional
   Ventricular
Parasystole
Capture beat
Reciprocal beat
Better atrioventricular conduction (e.g., 3:2), interrupting
   poorer (e.g., 2:1)

Supernormal conduction during advanced atrioventricular
    block
Rhythm resumption after inapparent bigeminy

Bradycardia (<60 beats/min)
Sinus bradycardia
Atrioventricular junctional rhythm
Sinus arrhythmia
Wandering atrial pacemaker
Sinoatrial block (second and third degree)
Sinus pause or arrest
Nonconducted atrial or ventricular bigeminy
Hypersensitive carotid sinus syndrome
Atrioventricular block (second and third degree)
Supraventricular tachyarrhythmias with high-grade atrioven-
    tricular block (rare)
Escape rhythms (resulting from bradycardia of any cause)
    Atrioventricular junctional
    Idioventricular
Sick sinus syndrome

References
1. Marriott, HJL: See Bibliography, 6.
2. Shander, D: Palpitation and Disorders of the Heartbeat, p.
    117. See Bibliography, 4.
3. Zipes, DP: Specific Arrhythmias; Diagnosis and
    Treatment, p. 646. See Bibliography, 1.

Tachycardia (Ventricular Rate >100 Beats/Min)

	Atrial rate	Ventricular rate	Ventricular response to carotid sinus massage
NORMAL QRS (<0.10 SEC)			
Regular rhythm			
Sinus tachycardia	100–200 (usually <160)	100–200 (usually <160)	Gradual slowing with return to previous rate. No effect or abrupt termination.
Atrioventricular (AV) nodal re-entry	140–250	140–250	May abruptly and transiently decrease ventricular rate; generally contraindicated.
Atrial tachycardia with block	140–250	Variable (usually 75–200)	May transiently slow ventricular rate, revealing flutter waves.
Atrial flutter	250–320	Variable (usually 75–175)	May transiently slow ventricular rate, revealing flutter waves.
Paroxysmal AV junctional tachycardia	100–180	100–180	No effect or abrupt termination.
Nonparoxysmal AV junctional tachycardia	Depends on atrial mechanism	65–130	No effect or gradual slowing with return to previous rate; generally contraindicated.
Reciprocating tachycardias using an accessory Wolff-Parkinson-White syndrome pathway	150–250	150–250	No effect or abrupt termination.
Ventricular tachycardia	Equal to or less than ventricular rate	60–250 (usually >150 and may be slightly irregular)	Atrial rate may slow; no effect on ventricular rate.
Irregular rhythm			
Atrial fibrillation	350–600	Variable	Transient decrease in ventricular rate.
Paroxysmal atrial tachycardia with variable block	140–250	Variable	May abruptly and transiently decrease ventricular rate; generally contraindicated.
Atrial flutter with variable block	250–300	Variable	Transient slowing of ventricular rate, revealing flutter waves.
Multifocal atrial tachycardia	100–200	100–200	No effect or gradual slowing.

Causes of the Eight Basic Rhythm Patterns

Regular rhythm at normal rates
    Normal sinus rhythm
    Accelerated junctional rhythm
    Accelerated idioventricular rhythm
    Atrial flutter with 4:1 conduction
    Atrial tachycardia with block
Early beats
    Extrasystole
    Parasystole
    Capture beats
    Intermittent improved conduction during heart block
    Rhythm resumption after inapparent bigeminy
Pauses
    Nonconducted premature atrial contractions (PACs) (most
        common)
    Second-degree atrioventricular (AV) block (types I
        and II)
    Second-degree sinoatrial (SA) exit block
    Concealed conduction
    Concealed junctional extrasystoles
Bradycardia
    Sinus bradycardia
    Nonconducted atrial bigeminy
    Second- and third-degree AV block
    Second- and third-degree SA block
Bigeminy
    PACs and premature ventricular contractions (PVCs)
    3:2 SA and AV block
    Atrial tachycardia or flutter with alternate 4:1 and 2:1
        conduction
    Nonconducted atrial trigeminy
    Reciprocal beating
    Concealed junctional extrasystoles
Chaos
    Atrial fibrillation
    Atrial flutter with variable conduction
    Multifocal atrial tachycardia
    Wandering pacemaker
    Multifocal PVCs
    Parasystoles
    Combinations of the above
Regular tachycardia
    Sinus tachycardia
    Paroxysmal atrial tachycardia

Atrial flutter
Ectopic atrial tachycardia
Junctional tachycardia
Ventricular tachycardia
Group beating
Nonconducted extrasystoles
SA nodal Wenckebach exit block
AV nodal Wenckebach block

Adapted from Marriott HJL: *Practical Electrocardiography*, 7/e.
Baltimore: Williams & Wilkins, 1983.

Differentiation of Aberrant Ventricular Condition from Ventricular Ectopy

Characteristics favoring aberrant ventricular conduction
Right bundle branch block with R' >R
Rate >170
Initial QRS vector same as conducted QRS
QRS duration <140 msec
Normal axis
Preceding P'
Ashman's phenomenon
Characteristics favoring ventricular ectopy
Left axis deviation
QRS >140 msec
Monophasic or diphasic in V1
Fusion or capture beats
Rate <170
Atrioventricular dissociation
R >R' in V1
Concordant precordial pattern

2-P. Electrocardiographic Abnormalities

QRS Interval, Prolonged
Bundle-branch blocks
Nonspecific intraventricular conduction delay
Aberrant ventricular conduction
Ectopic ventricular rhythm (e.g., ventricular parasystole)
Drug effect (e.g., quinidine or procainamide)
Electrolyte abnormalities (hyperkalemia, hypokalemia, hyper-
calcemia, hypermagnesemia)

Preexcitation (Wolff-Parkinson-White syndrome)
Left ventricular enlargement
Periinfarction block
Hypothermia

ST Segment Changes
Elevation
    Normal variant (e.g., early repolarization)
    Artifact
    Myocardial infarction
    Prinzmetal's angina
    Ventricular aneurysm
    Reciprocal changes
    Pericarditis
    Hyperkalemia (rarely)
    Bundle-branch block
    Acute cor pulmonale (e.g., pulmonary thromboembolism)
    Myocarditis
    Neoplastic heart disease
    Stroke
    Hypertrophic cardiomyopathy
    Hypothermia
    Cocaine abuse
Depression
    Nonspecific abnormality (e.g., anxiety, shock)
    Drugs
        Digitalis
        Tricyclic antidepressants
        Lithium
    Bundle-branch block
    Left or right ventricular strain
    Electrolyte abnormalities (hyperkalemia or hypokalemia)
    Subendocardial ischemia or infarction
    Mitral valve prolapse
    Tachycardia
    Myocarditis or cardiomyopathy
    Reciprocal changes
    Cerebral or subarachnoid injury
    Pancreatitis or other acute intraabdominal catastrophe
    Pulmonary thromboembolism
    Hypothyroidism

QT Interval
Prolonged
    Electrolyte abnormalities [hypocalcemia, hypokalemia,
            ("QU" prolongation)]

Complete heart block
Mitral valve prolapse
Left ventricular enlargement
Myocardial infarction and ischemia
Myocarditis and cardiomyopathy
Diffuse myocardial disease
Cerebral or subarachnoid injury, including surgical
Drugs (e.g., quinidine, procainamide, phenothiazines, sotalol,
     amiodarone, terfenadine, tricyclic antidepressants)
Hypothermia
Heritable anomaly
Alkalosis
Shortened
Electrolyte abnormalities (hypercalcemia, hyperkalemia,
     hypermagnesemia)
Digitalis
Acidosis

T-Wave Changes

Peaking
Normal variant
Nonspecific abnormality
Electrolyte abnormalities (hyperkalemia, hypocalcemia,
     hypomagnesemia)
Acute myocardial ischemia or infarction
Reciprocal effect in strictly posterior myocardial infarction
Left ventricular enlargement
Anemia
Cerebrovascular disease
Mitral or aortic regurgitation
Inversion
Normal
Juvenile T-wave pattern
Left bundle-branch block
Nonspecific abnormality
Myocardial ischemia or infarction
Myocarditis
Pericarditis
Ventricular strain
Acute or chronic cor pulmonale
Cerebral or subarachnoid injury
Drugs (e.g., quinidine, phenothiazines)
Electrolyte abnormalities (hypokalemia, hypomagnesemia)
Complete AV block
Vagotomy
After tachycardia

Q Waves, Abnormal

Myocardial infarction
Ischemia (transient)
Dextrocardia or dextroversion
Hypertrophic cardiomyopathy
Reversal of right and left arm leads (lead I)
Ventricular enlargement
Acute and chronic cor pulmonale (e.g., pulmonary embolism, chronic obstructive pulmonary disease)
Preexcitation (Wolff-Parkinson-White syndrome)
Cardiac surgery
Spontaneous pneumothorax (especially left)
Cardiomyopathy and myocarditis (e.g., hypertrophic cardiomyopathy; see 2-H)
Localized destructive myocardial disease (e.g., neoplasm)
Left bundle-branch block
Left anterior division block
Normal variant (rare)
Tachycardia (transitory)
Critical illness (e.g., pancreatitis, shock)

References

1. Friedman, p. 117. See Bibliography, 4.
2. Marriott, HJL: See Bibliography, 6.
3. Fisch C: Electrocardiography and Vectorcardiography, p. 108. See Bibliography, 1.
4. Fisch C: Electrocardiography, Exercise Stress Testing and Ambulatory Monitoring, p. 494. See Bibliography, 5.

2-Q. Cardiac Risk Index for Noncardiac Surgical Procedures

Computation of the Cardiac Risk Index

Criteria	"Points"
1. History	
a. Age >70 yr	5
b. MI in previous 6 mo	10
2. Physical examination	
a. S_3 gallop or JVD	11
b. Important VAS	3
3. Electrocardiogram	
a. Rhythm other than sinus or PACs on last preoperative ECG	7
b. >5 PVCs/min documented at any time before operation	7
4. General status: Po_2 <60 or Pco_2 >50 mm Hg, K <3.0 or HCO_3^- <20 mEq/L, BUN >50 or Cr >3.0 mg/dl, abnormal SGOT, signs of chronic liver disease, or patient bedridden from noncardiac causes	3
5. Operation	3
a. Intraperitoneal, intrathoracic, or aortic	3
b. Emergency	4
Total possible:	53

BUN, blood urea nitrogen; Cr, creatinine; ECG, electrocardiogram; HCO_3, bicarbonate; JVD, jugular vein distention; K, potassium; MI, myocardial infarction; PACs, premature atrial contractions; PVCs, premature ventricular contractions; SGOT, serum glutamic oxaloacetic transaminase; VAS, valvular aortic stenosis.

Adapted from Goldman L, Caldera DL, Nussbaum SR, et al: Multifactorial Index of Cardiac Risk in Non-Cardiac Surgical Procedures. *N Engl J Med* 297:848, 1977. By permission of the *New England Journal of Medicine*.

Cardiac Risk Index

Class	Point total	No (or only minor) complications[b] (N = 943)	Life-threatening complication[a] (N = 39)	Cardiac deaths (N = 19)
I (N = 537)	0–5	532 (99)	4 (0.7)	1 (0.2)
II (N = 316)	6–12	295 (93)	16 (5)	5 (2)
III (N = 130)	13–25	112 (86)	15 (11)	3 (2)
IV (N = 18)	>26	4 (22)	4 (22)	10 (56)

[a]Documented intraoperative or postoperative myocardial infarction, pulmonary edema, or ventricular tachycardia without progression to cardiac death.

[b]Figures in parentheses denote percentages.

From Goldman L, Caldera DL, Nussbaum SR, et al: Multifactorial Index of Cardiac Risk in Non-Cardiac Surgical Procedures. *N Engl J Med* 297:848, 1977. Reprinted by permission of the *New England Journal of Medicine*.

References
1. Goldman L: General Anesthesia and Non-Cardiac Surgery in Patients with Heart Disease, p. 1756. See Bibliography, 1.
2. Goldman L, Caldera DL, Nussbaum SR, et al: Multifactorial Index of Cardiac Risk in Non-Cardiac Surgical Procedures. *N Engl J Med* 297:845, 1977.
3. Margano DT, Goldman L: Preoperative Assessment of Patients with Known or Suspected Coronary Disease. *N Engl J Med* 333:1750, 1997.
4. American College of Cardiology, American Heart Association. Guidelines for Perioperative Cardiovascular Evaluation for Non-Cardiac Surgery. *Circulation* 95:1280–1317, 1996.

Bibliography

1. Braunwald E: *Heart Disease—A Test Book of Cardiovascular Medicine*. Philadelphia: WB Saunders, 1997.
2. Fauci AS, Braunwald E, Isselbacher KJ, et al (eds): *Harrison's Principles of Internal Medicine*, 14/e. New York: McGraw-Hill, 1998.
3. Friedman HH: *Diagnostic Electrocardiography and Vectorcardiography*, 3/e. New York: McGraw-Hill, 1984.
4. Friedman HH: *Problem-Oriented Medical Diagnosis*, 6/e. Philadelphia: Little, Brown and Company, 1996.
5. Kelley WN: *Textbook of Internal Medicine*, 3/e. Philadelphia: Lippincott–Raven, 1997.
6. Marriott HJL: *Practical Electrocardiography*, 8/e. Baltimore: Williams & Wilkins, 1988.

3 DRUGS

3-A. Bacterial Endocarditis Prophylaxis in Adults

CARDIAC CONDITIONS

Endocarditis Prophylaxis Recommended
  High Risk
    Prosthetic cardiac valves (bioprosthetic and homograft valves)
    Previous bacterial endocarditis (even without heart disease)
    Complex cyanotic congenital cardiac disease
    Surgically constructed systemic pulmonary shunts or conduits
  Moderate Risk
    Rheumatic and other acquired valvular dysfunction (even after valvular surgery)
    Hypertrophic cardiomyopathy (idiopathic hypertrophic subaortic stenosis)
    Mitral valve prolapse with valvular regurgitation and/or thickened leaflets
    Most other congenital cardiac malformations

Endocarditis Prophylaxis Not Recommended
  Isolated secundum atrial septal defect
  Surgical repair without residua beyond 6 mo of secundum atrial septal defect, ventricular septal defect, patent ductus arteriosus
  Previous coronary artery bypass graft surgery
  Mitral valve prolapse without valvular regurgitation

Physiologic, functional, or innocent heart murmurs
Previous Kawasaki's disease without valvular dysfunction
Previous rheumatic fever without valvular dysfunction
Cardiac pacemakers and implanted defibrillators

DENTAL OR SURGICAL PROCEDURES*

Endocarditis Prophylaxis Recommended
Dental procedures known to induce gingival or mucosal
    bleeding, including professional cleaning
Tonsillectomy and/or adenoidectomy
Surgical operations involving intestinal or respiratory
    mucosa
Bronchoscopy with a rigid bronchoscope
Sclerotherapy for esophageal varices
Esophageal dilation
Gallbladder surgery
Endoscopic retrograde cholangiography with biliary
    obstruction
Cystoscopy
Urethral dilation
Urethral catheterization, with urinary tract infection
Urinary tract surgery, with urinary tract infection
Prostatic surgery
Incision and drainage of infected tissue
Vaginal hysterectomy in high-risk patients
Vaginal delivery or abortion in the presence of infection
Manipulation of intrauterine device or dilation and curet-
    tage in the presence of infection

Endocarditis Prophylaxis Not Recommended
Dental procedures not likely to induce gingival bleeding
    (e.g., simple adjustment of orthodontic appliances
    or fillings above the gum line)
Injection of local intraoral anesthetic (except intraligamen-
    tary injections)
Shedding of primary teeth
Tympanostomy tube insertion
Endotracheal intubation
Bronchoscopy (flexible bronchoscope, with or without
    biopsy)
Cardiac catheterization, including angioplasty
Endoscopy, with or without gastrointestinal biopsy
Cesarean section
Transesophageal echocardiogram
Implanted cardiac pacemakers, defibrillators, or coronary
    stents

Incision or biopsy of surgically scrubbed skin
Circumcision
In the absence of infection: urethral catheterization, dilation and curettage, uncomplicated vaginal delivery, therapeutic abortion, sterilization procedures, or insertion or removal of intrauterine devices, laparoscopy

*For details, see reference 1.

References:
1. Kaschmer AW: Infective Endocarditis, p. 1097. See Bibliography, 6.
2. Dajani AS, et al: Prevention of Bacterial Endocarditis. *JAMA* 264:2919, 1990.
3. Dajani AS, et al: Prevention of Bacterial Endocarditis. *JAMA* 277:1794, 1997.
4. Durack DT: Prevention of Infective Endocarditis: *N Engl J Med* 332:38, 1995.

3-B. Prophylactic Regimens (in Adults)

Procedure	Recommended treatment
DENTAL, ORAL, UPPER RESPIRATORY TRACT, OR ESOPHAGEAL PROCEDURES	
Standard	Amoxicillin, 2 g, p.o. 1 hr before procedure
For patients unable to take oral medication	Ampicillin, 2 g, i.v. (or i.m.) 30 min before procedure
For ampicillin/amoxicillin/penicillin-allergic patients	Clindamycin, 600 mg, p.o. 1 hr before procedure
	or
	Cephalexin* or Cefadroxil,* 2 g, p.o. 1 hr before procedure
	or
	Azithromycin, or Clarithromycin, 500 mg, p.o. 1 hr before procedure
For ampicillin/amoxicillin/penicillin–allergic patients, unable to take oral medication	Clindamycin, 600 mg, i.v. 30 min before procedure
	or
	Cefazolin,* 1.0 g, i.v. or i.m. 30 min before procedure
FOR GENITOURINARY AND GASTROINTESTINAL PROCEDURES	
High-risk patients	Ampicillin, 2 g, i.v. (or i.m.) plus gentamicin, 1.5 mg/kg, i.v. or i.m. (not to exceed 120 mg) 30 min before procedure; then amoxicillin, 1.0 g, p.o. 6 hr after initial dose or ampicillin, 1.0 g, i.v. or i.m.

High-risk patients allergic to amoxicillin/ampicillin	Vancomycin, 1 g, i.v. administered over 1 hr plus gentamicin, 1.5 mg/kg, i.v. or i.m. (not to exceed 120 mg) 1 hr before procedure
Moderate-risk patients	Amoxicillin, 2 gm, p.o. 1 hr before procedure or ampicillin, 2 g, i.v. or i.m. within 30 min of starting procedure
Moderate-risk patients allergic to ampicillin/amoxicillin	Vancomycin, 1.0 g, i.v. over 1–2 hr, complete infusion within 30 min of starting procedure

*Cephalosporins should not be used in patients with anaphylactic or urticarial reactions to penicillin.

Modified from Dajani AS, et al: Prevention of Bacterial Endocarditis. *JAMA* 277:1704, 1997; and Karchmer AW: Infective Endocarditis. p. 1077. See Bibliography. 6.

3-C. Guidelines for Tetanus Prophylaxis

History of tetanus immunization (doses)	Years since last dose	Clean minor wounds		All other wounds	
		Give Td[a]	Give TIG	Give Td	Give TIG[b]
Unknown or <3	—	Yes	No	Yes	Yes[c]
≥3	>10	Yes	No	Yes	No
≥3	5-10	No	No	Yes	No
≥3	<5	No	No	No[d]	No

[a]Adult-type tetanus and diphtheria toxoids (Td) for patients >6 yr old.
[b]Human tetanus immune globulin (TIG) is preferred given as 250 units i.m.
[c]500 units i.m. is preferred for highly tetanus-prone wounds.
[d]Unless primary immunization was "fluid" rather than absorbed vaccine.

References

1. Des Prez RM, Haas DW: Mycobacterium Tuberculosis, p. 2213. See Bibliography, 3.
2. American Thoracic Society and Centers for Disease Control and Prevention: Control of Tuberculosis in the United States. *Am Rev Respir Dis* 146:1623, 1992.
3. Treatment of Tuberculosis and Tuberculosis Infection in Adults and Children. *Am J Respir Crit Care Med* 149:1359, 1994.

3-D. Recommendations for Isoniazid Prophylaxis[a]

Risk group	Age	Tuberculin reaction (mm)	Duration of treatment (mo)
HIV-infected persons	All	>5[b]	12
Close contacts of tuberculosis patients[c]	All	>5	6 (9 for children)
Persons with fibrotic lesions on chest radiography	All	>5	12
Recently infected persons	All	>10	6
Persons with high-risk medical conditions[d]	All	>10	6–12
High-incidence group[e]	<35 yr	>10	6
Low-incidence group	<35 yr	>15	6

[a]1. Before isoniazid chemoprophylaxis is begun, it is essential to exclude active infection (for which single-drug therapy is inadequate). 2. If isoniazid resistance is suspected, an alternative prophylactic regimen may be appropriate. 3. Isoniazid is contraindicated in the presence of active liver disease.

[b]Anergic human immunodeficiency virus (HIV)–infected persons with an estimated risk of M. tuberculosis infection of 10% may also be considered candidates.

[c]Tuberculin-negative contacts, especially children, should receive prophylaxis for 2 or 3 months after contact ends and should then be retested with purified protein derivative. Those whose results remain negative should discontinue prophylaxis.

[d]Includes diabetes mellitus, prolonged therapy with systemic glucocorticoids, other immunosuppressive therapy, some hematologic and reticuloendothelial diseases, injection drug use (with HIV seronegativity), end-stage renal disease, and clinical situations associated with rapid weight loss, or chronic undernutrition.

[e]Includes persons born in high-prevalence counties, members of medically underserved low-income populations, and residents of long-term-care facilities.

References

1. George WC, Feinegold SM: Clostridial Infection, p. 1673. See Bibliography, 2.
2. Brand DA, et al: Adequacy of Antitetanus Prophylaxis in Six Hospital Emergency Rooms. *N Engl J Med* 309:636, 1983.
3. Greenstein WA, Hinman AR, Bart KJ, et al, p. 2117. See Bibliography, 3.
4. Centers for Disease Control and Prevention: Diphtheria, Tetanus, and Pertussis: Recommendations for Vaccine Use and Other Preventative Measures. Recommendations for the Immunization Practices Advisory Committee (ACIP). *MMWR Morb Mortal Wkly Rep* 40:1–28, 1991.

Modified from Recommendations of the American Thoracic Society and the Centers for Disease Control and Prevention, 1994.

3-E. Selected Venereal Diseases: Current Treatment Recommendations

Gonorrhea

Diagnosis	Recommended treatment
Gonococcal infection in men and women	Ceftriaxone, 125 mg, i.m. or Ciprofloxacin,[a] 500 mg, once p.o. or Ofloxacin,[a] 400 mg, once p.o. or Cefixime,[b] 400 mg, once p.o. or Spectinomycin,[c] 2 g, i.m. once Concomitant *Chlamydia* therapy is recommended: Azithromycin[a] 1 g, p.o. once or Doxycycline,[a] 100 mg, p.o. b.i.d. for 7 days or Ofloxacin,[a] 300 mg, b.i.d. for 7 days or Erythromycin stearate, 500 mg, q.i.d. for 7 days

Pelvic inflammatory disease
  Hospitalized patients (at least 4 days
  of i.v. and 14 days of total therapy)
	Cefoxitin, 2 g, i.v. q6h, or cefotetan, 2 g, i.v. q12h, plus doxycycline,[a]
	  100 mg, i.v. q12h, followed by doxycycline,[a] 100 mg, p.o. b.i.d. to
	  complete 14 days of therapy or
	Clindamycin, 900 mg, i.v. q8h plus gentamicin, 2 mg/kg, i.v. once, followed
	  by 1.5 mg/kg i.v. q8h[d] followed by doxycycline,[a] 100 mg, p.o. b.i.d. to
	  complete 14 days of therapy

Outpatients	Cefoxitin, 2 g, i.m. once plus Probenecid, 1 g, p.o. once or Ceftriaxone, 250 mg, i.m. once Either regimen followed by doxycycline, 100 mg, b.i.d. p.o. for 14 days or *Continued*

3-E. Selected Venereal Diseases: Current Treatment Recommendations (continued)

Diagnosis	Recommended treatment
	Ofloxacin,[a] 400 mg, p.o. b.i.d. for 14 days plus Metronidazole, 500 mg, b.i.d. for 14 days or Clindamycin, 450 mg, p.o. q.i.d. for 14 days
Disseminated gonococcal infection (arthritis-dermatitis syndrome)	Ceftriaxone, 1 g, i.v. or i.m. q24h × 7–10 days or Cefotaxime, 1 g, i.v. q8h × 7–10 days or Ceftizoxime, 1 g, i.v. q8h × 7–10 days In β-lactam allergic patients, spectinomycin, 2 g, i.m. q12h Reliable patients, after symptoms resolve, can complete 10 days therapy with: Ciprofloxacin,[a] 500 mg, b.i.d. or Cefixime,[b] 400 mg, p.o. b.i.d. Concomitant *Chlamydia* therapy should be prescribed
Chlamydia trachomatis Nongonococcal urethritis in adults	Azithromycin, 1 g, p.o. single dose Doxycycline,[a] 100, g, p.o. b.i.d. for 7 days Tetracycline,[a] 500 mg, p.o. q.i.d. for 7 days Erythromycin stearate, 500 mg, p.o. q.i.d. for 7–21 days
In pregnancy	Erythromycin stearate, 500 mg, q.i.d. × 7 days or Amoxicillin, 500 mg, t.i.d. × 10 days

[a]Contraindicated in pregnancy.
[b]Efficacy in pregnancy not established.
[c]Ineffective in pharyngeal infection. Recommended only for use during pregnancy in patients allergic to β-lactams.
[d]Dose modification may be required in renal insufficiency.

Syphilis

Diagnosis/stage	Recommended treatment[a]	
	Non-penicillin-allergic	Penicillin-allergic
Primary, secondary, or early latent	Penicillin G benzathine, 2.4 million units i.m. (one-half in each hip) as single dose	Erythromycin stearate, 500 mg p.o. q.i.d., or doxycycline,[b] 100 mg p.o. b.i.d. for 14 days
Late-latent, latent of undetermined duration, cardiovascular, benign tertiary	Penicillin G benzathine, 2.4 million units i.m. once a week for 3 weeks	Erythromycin stearate or doxycycline,[b] 100 mg p.o. b.i.d. for 30 days
Neurosyphilis	Aqueous crystalline penicillin G, 2.4 million units i.v. q4h for 10–14 days; or penicillin G procaine, 2.4 million units i.m. q.d., and probenecid 500 mg p.o. q.i.d., both for 10–14 days	Skin test for penicillin allergy; desensitize if necessary
In pregnancy	Same as for nonpregnant, according to stage	Skin test for penicillin allergy; desensitize if necessary

[a]In HIV-positive patients, modified treatment regimens may be indicated.
[b]Contraindicated in pregnancy.

Continued

3-E. Selected Venereal Diseases (continued)

Herpes Simplex

Diagnosis	Recommended treatment
Primary genital	Acyclovir, 400 mg, p.o. t.i.d. for 7–10 days
Primary proctitis	Acyclovir, 800 mg, p.o. t.i.d. for 7–10 days
Recurrent	Acyclovir, 400 mg, p.o. t.i.d. for 5 days
Severe	Acyclovir, 5 mg/kg, i.v. q8h for 5–7 days
Prevention	Acyclovir, 400 mg, p.o. b.i.d.

References

1. Drugs for Sexually Transmitted Diseases. *Med Lett Drugs Ther* 37:117, 1995.
2. Tramont ED: Treponema Pallidum (Syphilis), p. 2117. See Bibliography, 3.

3-F. Common Drugs Requiring Dosage Adjustment in Renal Failure

Antibiotics
Acyclovir
Amantadine
Aminoglycosides (e.g., tobramycin)
Amphotericin
Ampicillin
Aztreonam
Cephalosporins (except cefoperazone, ceftriaxone)
Chloroquine
Cidofovir
Ciprofloxacin and all quinolones
Clarithromycin
Cycloserine
Delavirdine
Didanosine
Doxycycline
Ethambutol
Famciclovir
Fluconazole
5-Fluorocytosine
Foscarnet
Ganciclovir
Imipenem

Indinavir
Itraconazole
Isoniazid (especially slow acetylators)
Lamivudine
Meropenem
Metronidazole
Nalidixic acid
Nevirapine
Nitrofurantoin
Ofloxacin
Penicillins (except cloxacillin, dicloxacillin, nafcillin, oxacillin)
Pentamidine
Pyrazinamide
Ribavirin
Rimantadine
Stavudine
Sulfamethoxazole-trimethoprim
Sulfisoxazole
Terbinafine
Tetracyclines (except minocycline)
Trimethoprim
Valacyclovir
Vancomycin
Zalcitabine
Zidovudine

Analgesics
Acetaminophen
Aspirin
Butorphanol
Codeine
Fentanyl
Meperidine
Methadone
Morphine
Pentazocine
Phenazopyridine (Pyridium)
Propoxyphene (Darvon)

Sedatives and Psychiatric Drugs
Buspirone
Chlordiazepoxide (Librium)
Chloral hydrate
Ethchlorvynol
Glutethimide (Doriden)

Lithium carbonate
Lorazepam
Meprobamate
Methaqualone
Midazolam
Venlafaxine

Cardiovascular Drugs
Acebutolol
Acetazolamide
Amiloride
Atenolol
Betaxolol
Bretylium
All angiotensin-converting enzyme inhibitors (except fosinopril)
Digitoxin (for creatinine clearance <10 mL/min)
Digoxin
Disopyramide (Norpace)
Ethacrynic acid
Flecainide
Guanethidine
Hydralazine
Methyldopa
Mexiletine
Moricizine
Nadolol
Nitroprusside
Procainamide
Propafenone
Reserpine
Sotalol
Spironolactone
Thiazides
Tocainide
Triamterene
Verapamil

Antineoplastic and Immunosuppressive Drugs
Azathioprine
Bleomycin
Cisplatin
Cyclophosphamide
Daunorubicin
Doxorubicin

Etoposide
Fludarabine
Hydroxyurea
Melphalan
Methotrexate
Mitomycin C
Nitrosourea
Plicamycin
Streptozotocin

Arthritic Drugs

Acetaminophen
Allopurinol
Aspirin
Colchicine
Diflunisal
Gold
Ketorolac
Penicillamine
Phenylbutazone
Probenecid
Sulfinpyrazone
Sulindac

Anticonvulsants

Carbamazepine (Tegretol)
Ethosuximide
Phenobarbital
Primidone
Trimethadione
Valproic acid

Miscellaneous Agents

Baclofen
Cetirizine
Cimetidine
Clofibrate
Diphenhydramine (Benadryl)
Famotidine
Fexofenadine
Gallamine (Flaxedil)
Gemfibrozil
Hypoglycemic agents

    Acetohexamide (Dymelor)
    Chlorpropamide (Diabinese)
    Insulin
    Metformin
    Tolbutamide (Orinase)
Magnesium antacids
Metoclopramide
Neostigmine
Nicotinic acid
Nizatidine
Pancuronium
Pravastatin
Propylthiouracil
Ranitidine
Simvastatin
Terbutaline (especially parenteral)

References

1. Huey WY, Coyne DW: Dosage Adjustments of Drugs in Renal Failure, p. 549. See Bibliography, 1.
2. Swan SK, Bennett WM: Use of Drugs in Patients with Renal Failure, p. 2963. See Bibliography, 5.

3-G. Guidelines for Intravenous Aminophylline Therapy*

Loading Dose

	Dose (mg/kg)[a]
No known theophylline ingestion in past 24–48 hr	5–6 mg/kg over 15–30 min[b]
Theophylline ingested within past 48 hr	0–4 mg/kg over 15–30 min[c]
Poor clinical response to initial loading dose and no clinical signs of toxicity, or theophylline blood level <15 µg/mL	Additional 1–3 mg/kg over 15–30 min

[a]Based on ideal body weight.
[b]To raise serum level by 10 µg/mL.
[c]Therapy is guided by theophylline blood level, if available.

Maintenance Dose (Continuous Infusion)*

	Dose (mg/kg/hr)[a,b]
Children >9 yr old and adult smokers <55 yr old	0.50–0.90
Adult nonsmokers	0.40–0.60
Severe airway obstruction	0.40
Mild-to-moderate heart failure	<0.40
Severe heart failure	<0.20
Pneumonia	0.20–0.40
Liver dysfunction with serum bilirubin <1.5 mg/dL and serum albumin >2.9 g/dL	<0.45
Liver dysfunction with serum bilirubin >1.5 mg/dL and/or serum albumin <2.9 g/dL	<0.20

[a]Adolescents and/or smokers generally metabolize theophylline more rapidly and often receive higher doses.

[b]Patients taking propranolol, isoniazid, calcium channel blockers, mexiletine, pentoxifylline, caffeine, erythromycin, clarithromycin, tacrine, fluvoxamine, disulfiram, interferon, human recombinant alpha-A, methotrexate, mexiletine, ticlopidine, cimetidine, troleandomycin (Tao), thiabendazole, mebendazole, ciprofloxacin, allopurinol, oral contraceptives, norfloxacin, enoxacin, or ofloxacin metabolize theophylline more slowly and may require a reduction in dosage. Patients taking phenytoin, phenobarbital, carbamazepine, moricizine, aminoglutethimide, furosemide, or rifampin may require an increase in dosage.

References

1. Hendeles L, Weinberger M: Poisoning Patients with Intravenous Theophylline (editorial). *Am J Hosp Pharm* 37:49, 1980.
2. Powell JR, et al: Theophylline Disposition in Acutely Ill Hospitalized Patients. *Am Rev Respir Dis* 118:229, 1978.
3. Hendeles L, Weinberger M, Bighley L: Disposition of Theophylline after a Single Intravenous Infusion of Aminophylline. *Am Rev Respir Dis* 118–197, 1978.
4. *Physicians' Desk Reference*. Montvale, NJ: Medical Economics Data, 1998, p. 1333.

*Serum theophylline determinations after 12–36 hr of continuous aminophylline infusion are useful.

3-H. Glucocorticoid Preparations

USP name	Trade name	Tablet size (mg)	Relative anti-inflammatory potency	Relative mineralocorticoid potency	Approximate equivalent dosage (mg)	Biological half-life (hr)[a]
Short-acting						
Hydrocortisone (cortisol)	Hydrocortone, Solu-Cortel[b]	5, 10, 20	1.0	1.0	20.0	8–12
Cortisone		5, 10, 20	0.8	0.8	25.0	8–12
Intermediate-acting						
Prednisone	Deltasone	1, 2.5, 5, 10	4.0	0.8	5.0	12–36
Methylprednisolone	Medrol, Solu-Medrol[b]	2, 4, 8, 16, 24, 32	5.0	0.5	4.0	12–36
Triamcinolone	Aristocort, Aristospan[b]		5.0	0	4.0	12–36

Long-acting						
Dexamethasone	Decadron, Dalalone[b]	0.25, 0.5, 0.75, 1.5, 4	25	0	0.75	36–72
Betamethasone	Celestone	0.6	25	0	0.60	36–72

[a] Apply to only oral and intravenous routes of administration.
[b] Parenteral form.
Modified from Dayogo-Jack S: Mineral and Metabolic Bone Disease, p. 459. See Bibliography, 1.

References

1. Shimmer PP, Parker KL: Adrenocorticotrophic Hormone, Adrenocortical Steroids and Their Synthetic Analogs; Inhibitor of the Synthesis and Actions of Adrenocortical Hormones, p. 1459. See Bibliography, 4.
2. Axelrod L: Glucocorticoid Therapy. Medicine 55:39, 1976.

3-I. Hypoglycemic Agents

Characteristics of Commonly Used Insulin Preparations*

Classification	Insulin preparation	Onset	Action Peak	Duration (hr)
Rapid-acting	Regular	i.v.: Immediate	15–30 min	2
		i.m.: 5–30 min	30–60 min	2–4
		s.c.: 15–60 min	2–6 hr	4–12
	Semilente	s.c.: 30–60 min	3–10 hr	8–18
	Lispro	s.c.: 15–30 min	1–2 hr	3–5
Intermediate-acting	Neutral protamine Hagedorn	s.c.: 1.5–4 hr	6–16 hr	12–24
	Lente	s.c.: 1–4 hr	6–16 hr	12–28
Long-acting	Protamine zinc insulin (PZI)	s.c.: 3–8 hr	14–26 hr	24–40
	Ultralente (bovine)	s.c.: 3–8 hr	8–28 hr	24–40
	Ultralente (human)	s.c.: 3–8 hr	4–10 hr	9–36
Mixed insulin	Novolin 70/30	30 min	2–12 hr	24

*Activity may be prolonged in renal failure.
Modified from Orland MJ: Diabetes Mellitus, p. 396. See Bibliography, 1.

Oral Hypoglycemic Agents

Type	Available form (mg)	Total daily dosage range (mg)	Duration of action (hr)	Dose given	Excretion
Sulfonylureas*					
Tolbutamide (Orinase)	250, 500	500–3,000	6–12	b.i.d.–t.i.d.	Renal
Chlorpropamide (Diabinese)	100, 250	100–500	up to 90	q.d.–b.i.d.	Renal
Tolazamide (Tolinase)	100, 250, 500	100–1,000	12–24	q.d.–b.i.d.	Renal
Glipizide (Glucotrol)	5, 10	5–40	12–24	q.d.–b.i.d.	Renal 80%, bile 20%
Glipizide GITS	5	5–20	24–36	q.d.	Renal
Glyburide (DiaBeta, Micronase)	1.25–2.5	2.5–20	24–60	q.d.–b.i.d.	Renal 50%, bile 50%
Glyburide micronized	5.0 0.75	0.75–12	24–60	q.d.–b.i.d.	Renal 50%, bile 50%
Acetohexamide (Dymelor)	250, 750	250–1,500	12–24	q.d.–b.i.d.	Renal
Glimepiride (Amaryl)	1	1–8	24–60	q.d.	Renal 80%, bile 20%
Biguanide					
Metformin (Glucophage)	500, 850	500–3,000	12–24	q.d.–t.i.d.	Renal
α-Glucosidase inhibitor					
Acarbose (Precose)	25	75–300	2–6	t.i.d.	Largely not absorbed
Thiazolidinedione					
Troglitazone (Rezulin)	200	200–600	12–24	q.d.	Non-renal, likely significant, hepatic metabolism
Rosiglitazone maleate (Avandia)	2, 4, 8	4–8	12–24	q.d.–b.i.d.	Hepatic
Pioglitazone	15, 30, 45	15–45	24–36	q.d.	Hepatic

*Activity is prolonged in hepatic and renal failure.
Modified from Orland MJ: Diabetes Mellitus, p. 396. See Bibliography, 1.

Factors Causing Hyperglycemia in Diabetics
Weight gain or increased carbohydrate ingestion
Intravenous carbohydrate infusion (e.g., hyperalimentation)
Pubertal growth
Pregnancy
Nonuse or incorrect use of insulin
Infection or inflammation
Ketoacidosis
Emotional stress
Other acute stress (e.g., myocardial infarction, pancreatitis,
surgery)
Endocrinopathies
   Hyperthyroidism
   Pheochromocytoma
   Hyperadrenocorticism
   Profound hyperlipidemia
   Primary hyperparathyroidism
   Acromegaly
Decreased activity or exercise
Pancreatic disease or resection
Drug-induced pancreatic islet cell destruction (e.g., strepto-
zocin, pentamidine isethionate)
Hypokalemia
Hypomagnesemia
Drugs
   Nicotinic acid
   HIV protease inhibitors
   Diazoxide
   Sympathomimetics
   Glucocorticoids
   Phenytoin
   Thyroid hormone preparations
   Diuretics
   Oral contraceptives and other estrogens
Change in oral hypoglycemic therapy
Insulin or insulin-receptor antibodies
Insulin-resistant states

Factors Causing Hypoglycemia in Diabetics
Weight reduction or decreased carbohydrate ingestion
Decreased intravenous carbohydrate infusion
Increased activity
Overdose of insulin and/or sulfonylurea therapy
Drug interactions with sulfonylurea therapy
   Salicylates
   Clopidogrel

> Pentamidine
> Quinine
> Propranolol
> Sulfonamides

Renal insufficiency
Alcohol ingestion
Hypothyroidism
Hypoadrenocorticism
Decreased dosage or discontinuation of drugs (e.g., glucocorticoids, diuretics, thyroid hormone preparations)
Intercurrent processes causing hypoglycemia (e.g., insulinoma; see 4-V)

References
1. Orland MJ: Diabetes Mellitus and Related Disorders, p. 396. See Bibliography, 1.
2. Smith, RJ: Approach to the Patient with Hypoglycemia, p. 2166. See Bibliography, 2.

3-J. Selected Intravenous Vasoactive Drugs

Drug	Common preparations	Dosage	Comments
Epinephrine	5 mg/500 mL	Initial dose: 1–4 µg/min; titrate to effect.	Vasoconstrictor arrhythmias.
Amrinone (Inocor)	1 amp = 100 mg; dilute to 1–3 mg/mL concentration in saline solution; do not use dextrose	Initial dose: 0.75 mg/kg over 2–3 min and then infuse continuously 5–15 µg/kg/min.	Side effects: thrombocytopenia, gastrointestinal upset, fever, myalgia, hepatic dysfunction, ventricular irritability, and hypotension.
Milrinone (Primacor)	40 mg in 200 mL 5% D5W or NS	Initial dose: 50 µg/kg slow i.v.p. over 10 min and then infuse continuously 0.375–0.750 µg/kg/min; titrate to effect.	Side effects: hypertension, ventricular arrhythmias, headaches.
Sodium nitroprusside (Nipride)	1 amp = 50 mg; add 50 mg to 250 mL 5% D5W only	Initial dose: 0.3–5 µg/kg/min; titrate to effect only or maximum of 10 µg/kg/min; average effective dose is 3 µg/kg/min.	Infusion apparatus must be shielded from light; infusion pump is required; total dose >3 mg/kg may be associated with toxicity, especially when renal insufficiency is present.
Nitroglycerine	Usually 1 amp = 50 mg; add 50 mg to 250 mL 5% D5W or NS; follow supplier's recommendations	Initial dose: 3–10 µg/min/increase by 5–10 mg/min every 3–5 min until response seen. Usual maximum dose: 300 µg/min.	Use glass bottles or polyolefin containers and nonabsorbing tubing. Treat hypotension with volume and cessation of infusion.

Bretylium (Bretylol)	1 amp = 500 mg; add 2 g to 500 mL 5% D5W or NS	For ventricular tachycardia, 5–10 mg/kg (undiluted) over 10 min then infuse continuously 1–4 mg/min.	Hypotension and/or arrhythmias may be provoked.
Procainamide (Pronestyl)	10 mL vial = 1,000 mg; 2 mL vial = 1,000 mg; add 2 g to 500 mL 5% D5W or NS	Loading dose: <17 mg/kg i.v.p.b. at <50 mg/min; then infuse continuously 1–5 mg/min.	Hypotension is main toxicity.
Lidocaine (Xylocaine)	1 amp = 50 or 100 mg; premix 2 g in 500 mL 5% D5W	Initial dose: 50–100 mg i.v.p.; may repeat 0.5 mg/kg Q 10 min to a total of 3 mg/kg, then infuse continuously 1–4 mg/min.	No more than 200–300 mg of lidocaine should be administered during a 1 hr period. Usual toxicity is convulsions and confusion.
Amiodarone (Cordarone)	Dilute in D5W only	Loading dose: 150 mg over 10 min (may repeat), then 1 mg/min for 6 hr, then 0.5 mg/min continuously.	Nausea can occur with loading. Sinus brachycardia and AV block can occur.
Esmolol (Brevibloc)	Mix 2.5 mg in 250 mL D5W or NS	Initial dose: 500 µg/kg over 1 min then infuse at 50 µg/kg/min.	Toxicity includes hypotension, heart block, heart failure, bronchospasm.
Diltiazem (Cardizem)	250 mg/250 mg (1 mg/mL)	5–20 mg i.v. bolus initially then infuse at 5–20 mg/hr and titrate to effect.	Hypotension. Bradycardia.

Continued

3–J. Selected Intravenous Vasoactive Drugs (continued)

Drug	Common preparations	Dosage	Comments
Ibutilide (Corvert)	1 mg mix in 50 cc D5W or undiluted 1 mg/10 cc	1 mg i.v.p.b. over 10 min may repeat × 1 (if weight <60 kg use 0.01 mg/kg).	5% risk of serious proarrhythmias.
Nicardipine (Cardene)	Mix 25 mg in 250 cc NS or D5W	Infuse at 2–15 mg/hr.	Hypotension, headache.

AV, atrioventricular; D5W, dextrose 5% in water; NS, normal solution.

References

1. Botteron GW, Smith JM: Cardiac Arrhythmias, p. 130. See Bibliography, 1.
2. Carey CF, Schaiff AA: Intravenous Admixture, Preparation and Administration Guide, p. 546. See Bibliography, 1.

3-K. Drug and Disease Interactions with Warfarin (Coumadin)

Increased Prothrombin Time
Acetaminophen
Age
Alcohol*
Allopurinol
Aminoglycoside antibiotics (oral)
Amiodarone
Anabolic steroids
Azithromycin
Bromelains
Cancer
Cephalosporins (parenteral)
Chloral hydrate*
Chlorpropamide
Cholestyramine*
Chymotrypsin
Cimetidine
Ciprofloxacin
Clarithromycin
Clofibrate
Collagen vascular disease
Congestive heart failure
Cyclophosphamide*
Dextran
Dextrothyroxine
Diarrhea
Diazoxide
Diflunisal
Disopyramide
Disulfiram
Diuretics*
Doxycycline
Enoxacin
Erythromycin
Ethacrynic acid
Fenoprofen
Fever
Fluconazole
Fluorouracil
Fluoxetine
Gemfibrozil

Glucagon
Heparin
Hepatic disease
Hepatotoxic drugs
Hyperthyroidism
Hypoglycemic agents
Ibuprofen
Indomethacin
Influenza vaccine
Inhalation anesthetics
Isoniazid (600 mg daily)
Itraconazole
Ketoconazole
Ketoprofen
Lovastatin
Levamisole
Malnutrition
Mefenamic acid
Methimazole*
Methyldopa
Methylphenidate
Metronidazole
Miconazole
Monoamine oxidase inhibitors
Moricizine*
Nalidixic acid
Naproxen
Narcotics
Norfloxacin
Ofloxacin
Omeprazole
Oxyphenbutazone
Paroxetine
Penicillin
Pentoxifylline
Phenylbutazone
Phenytoin*
Piperacillin
Piroxicam
Prednisone
Propafenone
Propranolol
Propylthiouracil*
Pyrazolones
Quinidine
Quinine
Ranitidine*

Salicylates (>1 g daily)
Sertraline
Simvastatin
Steatorrhea
Streptokinase
Sulfinpyrazone
Sulfonamides
Sulindac
Tamoxifen
Tetracyclines
Thyroid preparations
Ticarcillin
Ticlopidine
Tissue plasminogen activator (t-PA)
Tolbutamide
Tolmetin
Tricyclic antidepressants
Trimethoprim-sulfamethoxazole
Unreliable prothrombin time (PT)/international normalized
      ratio (INR)
Urokinase
Valproic acid
Vitamin E
Vitamin K malabsorption or deficiency
Zafirlukast

*Can cause increased or decreased prothrombin time.

Decreased Prothrombin Time/International Normalized Ratio
Alcohol*
Aluminum hydroxide
Aminoglutethimide
Antihistamines
Azathioprine
Barbiturates
Carbamazepine
Chloral hydrate*
Chlordiazepoxide
Chlorthalidone
Cholestyramine*
Cyclophosphamide
Cyclosporine
Dicloxacillin
Diuretics*
Edema

Estrogens
Ethchlorvynol
Etretinate
Glucocorticoids
Glutethimide
Griseofulvin
Haloperidol
Hereditary resistance
Hyperlipidemia
Insecticides
Meprobamate
Methimazole
Moricizine*
Myxedema
Nafcillin
Nephrotic syndrome
Oral contraceptives
Paraldehyde
Pregnancy (mother only)
Prolonged hot weather
Primidone
Ranitidine*
Rifampin
Spironolactone
Sucralfate
Trazodone
Unreliable PT/INR
Vitamin C (high dose)
Vitamin K
Diet high in vitamin K

Reference

1. *Physicians' Desk Reference*. Montvale, NJ: Medical Economics Data, 1998, p. 866.

*Can cause increased or decreased prothrombin time.

3-L. Partial List of Drugs Used during Pregnancy

Type of medication	Safe to use in pregnancy[a]	Limited information, relatively safe[b]	Risks associated with use[c]	Avoid in pregnancy[d]
Analgesics	Acetaminophen	Hydromorphone[e] Codeine[e] Meperidine[e] Oxycodone with aspirin[e] Morphine[e]	Salicylates Ibuprofen Indomethacin	
Antibiotics	Ampicillin Erythromycin Penicillin Carbenicillin	Amikacin Amphotericin B Nitrofurantoin Ampicillin with sulbactam Amoxicillin with clavulanic acid Miconazole Aztreonam Ticarcillin Oxacillin Methicillin Cephalosporins Clindamycin Gentamicin Tobramycin	Chloramphenicol Metronidazole Isoniazid Streptomycin Sulfonamides Rifampin Trimethoprim Kanamycin	Chloroquine Ciprofloxacin Norfloxacin Tetracyclines
Anticoagulants		Dipyridamole Heparin		Warfarin

Continued

3-L. Partial List of Drugs Used During Pregnancy (continued)

Type of medication	Safe to use in pregnancy[a]	Limited information, relatively safe[b]	Risks associated with use[c]	Avoid in pregnancy[d]
Antiemetics		Meclizine Trimethobenzamide Metoclopramide	Thiethylperazine Prochlorperazine	
Antiepileptics		Ethosuximide	Clonazepam Phenytoin Valproic acid Primidone Phenobarbital	
Antihistamines	Tripelennamine		Brompheniramine Terfenadine Astemizole Diphenhydramine	Hydroxyzine
Antihypertensives		Hydralazine Methyldopa Clonidine Metoprolol Prazosin	Atenolol Nitroprusside Diazoxide Labetalol Timolol Propranolol Nadolol	Captopril Reserpine Enalapril Lisinopril
Asthma preparations		Beclomethasone Aminophylline	Albuterol Isoproterenol	

Category	Drugs
	Cromolyn sodium
	Terbutaline
	Ipratropium bromide
	Metaproterenol
Cardiac drugs	Digoxin, Procainamide, Atropine, Quinidine, Lidocaine, Verapamil, Disopyramide, Diltiazem, Nifedipine
Cough preparations	Terpin hydrate, Guaifenesin
Diuretics[f]	Furosemide, Bumetanide, Ethacrynic acid, Acetazolamide, Hydrochlorothiazide
Hypoglycemics[g]	Insulin, Chlorpropamide, Tolbutamide, Glyburide
Laxatives	Milk of magnesia, Psyllium, Docusate
Sedatives	Barbiturates, Benzodiazepines
Thyroid preparations	Thyroxine, Methimazole, Propylthiouracil, Iodide

Continued

3-L. Partial List of Drugs Used During Pregnancy (continued)

Type of medication	Safe to use in pregnancy[a]	Limited information, relatively safe[b]	Risks associated with use[c]	Avoid in pregnancy[d]
Other drugs	Ferrous sulfate Kaopectate Probenecid	Allopurinol Clofibrate H_2 antagonists	Glucocorticoids Amphetamines Ethylenediamine-tetraacetic acid	Antineoplastic agents Bromocriptine Lithium
	Antacids	Vaccines (influenza, polio, rabies, tetanus)	General anesthesia drugs Haloperidol Penicillamine Phenothiazines	Disulfiram Estrogens, diethyl-stilbestrol Isotretinoin Quinine Tricyclic antide-pressants Vaccines (rubella, mumps, measles, smallpox) Misoprostol

[a]No drug can be used with certainty that there will be no adverse effects.

[b]Many drugs in this column are new and data are limited, but no consistent adverse effect has been attributed to their use.

[c]These drugs have some associated risk when used in pregnancy. The potential benefit must be weighed against possible adverse effects.

[d]These drugs have been well documented to produce adverse fetal effects. They should not be used in pregnancy.

[e]Possible neonatal addiction and withdrawal may occur after long-term use. Neonatal depression may occur with intrapartum use. Diuretics can deplete maternal intravascular volume and, in rare instances, can be associated with neonatal thrombocytopenia. Diuretics are not indicated in pregnancy-induced hypertension as first-line agents.

[f]No place exists for oral hypoglycemic agents in the treatment of diabetes in pregnancy. Oral hypoglycemic agents have been associated with prolonged hypoglycemia in newborn infants; insulin and dietary control are indicated to bring blood sugar under rigid control.

From Nauser TD, McGahan MM: *Pregnancy and Medical Therapeutics*, p. 534. See Bibliography. 1.

Bibliography

1. Carey CF, Lee HH, Woeltje KF (eds): *The Washington Manual of Medical Therapeutics*, 29/e. Philadelphia: Lippincott–Raven, 1998, p. 130.
2. Kelly WN (ed): *Textbook of Internal Medicine*, 3/e. Philadelphia: Lippincott–Raven, 1997.
3. Mandell GL, et al. (eds): *Principles and Practice of Infectious Diseases*, 4/e. New York: Churchill Livingstone, 1997.
4. Hardman JG, Limbird LE: *Goodman & Gillman's The Pharmacological Basis of Therapeutics*. New York: McGraw-Hill, 1996.
5. Schrier RW, Gottschalk CW: *Diseases of the Kidney*, 6/e. Boston: Little, Brown and Company, 1997.
6. Braunwald E (ed): *Heart Disease*, 5/e. Philadelphia: WB Saunders, 1997.

4 ENDOCRINE/ METABOLIC SYSTEM

4-A. Hypothermia

Excessive Heat Loss
Cold-water immersion
Environmental exposure (especially in neonates, premature
        or low-birth-weight babies, the elderly, or persons
        who are unconscious, immobilized, drugged,
        under anesthesia, or exhausted)
    Accidental
    Iatrogenic
        Administration of cold blood or intravenous (i.v.) fluids
        Iced saline gastric lavage
        Peritoneal dialysis
Increased cutaneous blood flow
    Burns
    Erythrodermas (including toxic epidermal necrolysis and
        psoriasis)

Inadequate Heat Production
Altered thermoregulation
    Hypothalamic and central nervous system dysfunction
        (note: the hypothermia may be paroxysmal)
    Anorexia nervosa
    Brain tumors
    Cerebrovascular accidents, paralysis, paresis
    Episodic spontaneous hypothermia with hyperhidrosis
        (including those with agenesis of the corpus cal-
        losum—Shapiro's syndrome)

Head trauma
Other hypothalamic lesions (e.g., infarction, midbrain
lesions, sarcoidosis)
Seizure
Spinal cord transection above T1
Spontaneous periodic hypothermia (paroxysmal
hypothermia—nearly always with evidence of
injury to the preoptic area of the hypothalamus)
Wernicke's encephalopathy
Sepsis
Shock
Uremia
Decreased metabolism (especially in the elderly comatose)
Congestive heart failure
Endocrine disorders
Adrenal insufficiency
Diabetic ketoacidosis
Hypoglycemia
Hypopituitarism
Hypothyroidism
Gambian sleeping sickness
Hepatic failure
Malnutrition
Myocardial infarction
Prolonged cardiopulmonary resuscitation
Pancreatitis
Respiratory failure
Drugs
Antidepressants
Barbiturates
Benzodiazepines
Cancer chemotherapy
Cannabis
Clonidine
Ethanol
General anesthesia
Hypnotics
Lithium
Opiates
Phenothiazines
Sedatives
Tranquilizers

References
1. Petty KJ: Hypothermia, pp. 97–98. See Bibliography, 1.
2. Yoder E: Disorders Due to Heat and Cold, p. 503. See
Bibliography, 5.

4-B. Weight Gain

Cessation of cigarette smoking
Congenital disorders
    Alström syndrome
    Biemond syndrome
    Blount disease
    Börjeson's syndrome
    Carpenter's syndrome
    Cohen syndrome
    Laurence-Moon-Bardet-Biedl syndrome
    Prader-Willi syndrome
    Pseudohypoparathyroidism
Depression
Disturbances of hypothalamic satiety centers
    Encephalitis
    Trauma
    Tumors
Drugs
    Antidepressants
        Amitriptyline
        Amoxapine
        Desipramine
        Doxepin
        Imipramine
        Phenelzine
        Tranylcypromine
        Trazodone
    Antiepileptics
        Carbamazepine
        Valproate
    Antihypertensives
        Terazosin
    Glucocorticoids (pharmacologic doses)
    Megestrol acetate
    Oral contraceptives
    Phenothiazines
        Chlorpromazine
        Haloperidol
        Loxapine
        Mepazine
        Mesoridazine
        Perphenazine
        Prochlorperazine
        Promazine
        Thioridazine

Trifluoperazine
Endocrine disorders
Acromegaly
Cushing's syndrome
Hypothyroidism
Insulinoma
Exogenous obesity
Increased body fluid (see 2-B)

References

1. Foster DW: Gain and Loss in Weight, pp. 244–245. See Bibliography, 1.
2. Bray GA: Obesity, p. 454. See Bibliography, 1.

4-C. Weight Loss

Ankylosing spondylitis
Bilateral lesions of the lateral hypothalamus (hypothalamic anorexia)
Decreased food intake/malnutrition
Abdominal angina
Anorexia of aging
Chronic/recurrent nausea/vomiting
Dementia/Alzheimer's disease
Esophageal disease/dysphagia
Esophagitis
Neoplasm
Neuromuscular dysfunction
Reflux
Scleroderma
Stricture
Medications
Angiotensin-converting enzyme inhibitors (distortion of taste)
Antidepressants
Clonidine
Digoxin
Nonsteroidal antiinflammatory agents
Sedatives
Theophylline
Obstructive gastrointestinal disease (including pyloric obstruction due to chronic peptic ulcer disease)

Oral disease
    Loose dentures
    Poor or absent teeth
    Other oral diseases
Pain
Poor social situation
Postantrectomy (especially Billroth II) or gastrectomy
Poverty
Unpalatable diets
Endocrine disorders
    Adrenal insufficiency
    Diabetes mellitus
    Diabetic neuropathic cachexia
    Hypercalcemia
    Panhypopituitarism
    Pheochromocytoma
    Thyrotoxicosis
Extensive exercise
Infection, especially
    Amebic abscess
    Bacterial endocarditis
    Chronic suppurative pleuropulmonary disease (e.g.,
        emphysema)
    Cryptosporidiosis
    Fungal diseases
    Giardiasis
    Human immunodeficiency virus (HIV)
    Mycobacterium avium pulmonary infections
    Parasitic infestations
    Paraspinal/epidural abscess
    Tuberculosis
    Visceral leishmaniasis
Maldigestion/malabsorption
        Inflammatory bowel disease
        Pernicious anemia
Malignancy, especially
    Biliary
    Breast
    Gastrointestinal
    Glucagonoma
    Hepatic
    Leukemia
    Lymphoma
    Myeloma
    Pancreatic

    Pulmonary
    Somatostatinoma
Myelofibrosis
Myotonic dystrophy
Parkinson's disease
Pink disease (mercury poisoning in children)
Psychiatric disease
    Anorexia nervosa
    Anxiety disorders
    Bulimia
    Conversion disorders
    Depression
    Manipulative behaviors
    Psychosis/paranoia
    Schizophrenia
    Substance abuse
Severe chronic organ failure
    Heart failure (cardiac cachexia)
    Hepatic disease
    Pulmonary disease
    Renal failure
Systemic lupus erythematosus

References

1. Foster DW: Gain and Loss in Weight, p. 245. See Bibliography, 1.
2. Baron RB: Protein-Energy Malnutrition, p. 1154. See Bibliography, 5.

4-D. Thyrotoxicosis

Thyrotoxicosis with high or normal radioactive iodine uptake
Abnormal thyroid stimulator
    Human chorionic gonadotropin (HCG)
        Gestational thyrotoxicosis (with hyperemesis)
        Tumors secreting HCG
            Choriocarcinoma
            Hydatidiform mole
            Embryonal cell carcinoma of the testis
    Thyroid-stimulating hormone (TSH)
        Selective pituitary resistance to thyroid hormone
        TSH-secreting pituitary adenoma

Thyroid-stimulating immunoglobulins
  Graves' disease
  Hashitoxicosis
  Neonate of mother with Graves' disease
Autonomous thyroid function
  Constitutive activation of TSH receptors (autosomal
      dominant)
  Toxic adenoma
  Toxic multinodular goiter
Postaspiration thyrotoxicosis (after needle aspirate of
      thyroid cyst)
TSH hyperresponsiveness (autosomal dominant)

Thyrotoxicosis with a Low Radioactive Iodine Uptake

Excessive thyroidal production of thyroid hormone
  Iodine-induced thyrotoxicosis (the "jod-Basedow"
      phenomenon)
    Amiodarone
    Other iodine-containing drugs
    Iodine-containing x-ray contrast agents
Extrathyroidal sources of thyroid hormone
  Ectopic thyroid tissue
    Metastatic differentiated thyroid cancer
    Struma ovarii
  Hormone ingestion
    "Hamburger thyrotoxicosis"
    Iatrogenic
    Thyrotoxicosis factitia
Inflammation of the thyroid
  Drug-induced thyroiditis
    Amiodarone
    Interferon-α
    Interleukin-2
  Infarction of thyroid adenoma
  Postpartum thyroiditis
  Radiation thyroiditis
  Silent (painless) thyroiditis
  Subacute (DeQuervain's, granulomatous) thyroiditis
Postparathyroidectomy thyrotoxicosis (transient—2 weeks)

References

1. Burman KD: Hyperthyroidism, pp. 371–376. See
   Bibliography, 2.
2. Braverman LE, Utiger RD: Introduction to Thyrotoxicosis,
   pp. 522–524. See Bibliography, 4.

4-E. Hypothyroidism

Primary Hypothyroidism

Addison's disease (reversible hypothyroidism)
Addition of other drugs to levothyroxine therapy
    Aluminum hydroxide–containing antacids
    Bile acid sequestrants
    Ferrous sulfate
    Sertraline
    Sucralfate
Destruction of the thyroid gland
    External beam radiation therapy to the head/neck
    Radioactive iodine (may be transient)
    Replacement of thyroid tissue
        Infiltrative diseases
            Amyloidosis
            Chondrocalcinosis
            Cystinosis
            Hemochromatosis
            Histiocytosis X
            Riedel's thyroiditis
            Sarcoidosis and other granulomatous diseases
            Scleroderma
        Malignancies
            Lymphoma of the thyroid
            Metastatic nonthyroidal cancer
            Thyroid cancer
    Surgery (total or subtotal thyroidectomy) (may be transient)
    Thyroiditis
        Acute (suppurative) thyroiditis [bacterial, mycobacterial, fungal, parasitic, gummatous, Pneumocystis carinii infection in acquired immunodeficiency syndrome (AIDS)]
        Chronic
            Atrophic thyroiditis
            Hashimoto's thyroiditis
        Due to drug therapy
            Amiodarone
            Interferon-α
            Interleukin-2
            Lymphokine-activated killer cell therapy
        Transient
            Postpartum thyroiditis
            Silent (painless) thyroiditis
            Subacute (DeQuervain's, granulomatous) thyroiditis

Generalized resistance to thyroid hormone
Inhibition of thyroid hormone synthesis or accelerated disap-
        pearance from the circulation
    Exposure to exogenous goitrogens
        (see 4-I)
    Inherited defects of thyroid hormone synthesis
    Iodide deficiency
    Selenium deficiency (usually with concomitant iodide
        deficiency)
    Thyroid agenesis, dysgenesis, or ectopy
Thyroid growth-blocking antibodies
Transplacental passage of antithyroid drugs, chemicals, or
        agents
TSH hyporesponsiveness
    Abnormal G-protein (G_s activity)
        Pseudohypoparathyroidism type Ia
    TSH receptor abnormalities
    TSH receptor-blocking antibodies

Secondary (Pituitary) or Tertiary (Hypothalamic) Hypothyroidism*

    After withdrawal of thyroid hormone therapy in euthyroid
        patients (transient)
    Thyroid-releasing hormone deficiency or insensitivity
    TSH synthetic defect

References

1. Shapiro LE, Surks MI: Hypothyroidism, pp. 404–405. See
   Bibliography, 2.
2. Braverman LE, Utiger RD: Introduction to Hypothyroidism,
   pp. 736–737. See Bibliography, 4.

*See 4-5.

4-F. Serum Thyroxine

Elevated Total Thyroxine, but Normal Free Thyroxine

Increased affinity of serum binding proteins for thyroxine (T_4)
    Increased affinity of albumin for T_4
        Familial dysalbuminemic hyperthyroxinemia (total T_4
          and free T_4 index elevated, but free T_4 normal)
          (note: a familial dysalbuminemic hypertriiodothy-
          roninemia has also been described)

Increased affinity of transthyretin for T_4
    Familial increase in transthyretin binding (autosomal
        dominant) (total T_4 and free T_4 index elevated, but
        free T_4 normal)
Increased serum concentration of binding proteins for T_4
    Increased T_4-binding globulin (TBG) concentration
        Acute intermittent porphyria
        Estrogens (including oral contraceptives, but not usual in
          users of low-dose pills or transdermal estrogen)
        Drugs (small increases in TBG)
           Clofibrate
           Fluorouracil
           Opiates
           Perphenazine
           Tamoxifen
           HIV infection and AIDS
        Increased endogenous estrogen production
           Estrogen-secreting adrenal or testicular tumors
           Pregnancy
        Inherited increase in thyroid-binding globulin
        Liver disease
           Acute and chronic hepatitis
           Biliary cirrhosis
           Hepatoma
         Neonatal state
    Increased T_4 binding to autoantibodies to T_4
    Increased transthyretin concentration
        Pancreatic islet cell carcinoma

Elevated Total and Free Thyroxine
Thyrotoxicosis (see 4-D)
Iatrogenic (excessive doses of oral levothyroxine)
Amphetamines (large doses)
Antibodies that interfere with the thyroid hormone assay
    Human anti-mouse antibodies
Generalized resistance to thyroid hormone
High altitude
Inhibition of peripheral conversion of T_4 to triiodothyronine (T_3)
    5' deiodinase deficiency
    Drugs
        Amiodarone
        Oral cholecystographic agents
           Iobenzamic acid
           Iopanoic acid
           Sodium ipodate

Tyropanoate
Propranolol (high doses) (not atenolol or sotalol)
Neonatal period
Nonthyroidal illness (including acute psychiatric illness)

Decreased Total Thyroxine but Normal Free Thyroxine
Decreased levels of serum thyroid-binding proteins
    Acromegaly
    Cirrhosis
    Cushing's syndrome
    Drugs
        Androgens and anabolic steroids
        Asparaginase
        Chlorpropamide
        Colestipol combined with niacin
        Danazol
        Large doses of adrenocorticotropic hormone or gluco-
            corticoids (chronic)
        Salsalate
        Sulfonamides
    Inherited decrease in serum levels of TBG
        Malnutrition
    Protein loss (e.g., nephrotic syndrome)
    Nonthyroidal illness
    Testosterone-secreting adrenal or ovarian tumors
Decreased affinity of serum-binding proteins for T_4
    Decreased affinity of TBG for T_4
        Inherited TBG that has decreased affinity for T_4
        Nonthyroidal illness
    Decreased affinity of transthyretin for T_4
        Familial amyloidotic polyneuropathy
        Nonthyroidal illness
Displacement of T_4 from serum-binding sites
    Drugs
        Furosemide (acutely)
        Halofenate
        Heparin (acutely)
        Penicillin
        Phenylbutazone
        Salicylates (in high doses)
        Other nonsteroidal antiinflammatory drugs
            Fenclofenac
            Meclofenamic acid
            Mefenamic acid

Decreased Total and Free Thyroxine
Hypothyroidism (see 4-E)
Functional suppression of TSH secretion
    Drugs
        Dopamine
        Glucocorticoid excess or adrenocorticotrophic (ACTH)
            therapy
    Nonthyroidal illness (including anorexia nervosa)
Increased hepatic metabolism of T_4 (TSH usually remains
            normal)
    Carbamazepine
    Chlorpromazine
    Phenobarbital
    Phenytoin
    Reserpine
    Rifampin
Therapy with T_3 alone

References
1. Stockigt JR: Serum Thyrotropin and Thyroid Hormone
   Measurements and Assessment of Thyroid Hormone
   Transport, pp. 387–392. See Bibliography, 4.
2. Utiger RD: Physiology, Thyrotoxicosis, Hypothyroidism
   and the Painful Thyroid, pp. 521–529. See Bibliography, 6.

4-G. Serum Thyroid-Stimulating Hormone

Elevated Serum Thyroid-Stimulating Hormone
Primary hypothyroidism (see 4-E)
    Overt (low free T_4)
    Subclinical (normal free T_4)
Assay problems
    Assay variability
    Heterophile antibodies interfering with the TSH assay
Drugs
    Domperidone
    Metoclopramide
Pulsatile TSH secretion, nocturnal TSH surge
Recovery from nonthyroidal illness
Thyroid hormone resistance syndromes
TSH-secreting pituitary tumors

Suppressed Serum Thyroid-Stimulating Hormone
Thyrotoxicosis (see 4-D)
    Overt (low free T_4)

    Subclinical (normal free T_4)
    T_3 Toxicosis (with normal or low free T_4)
After treatment of thyrotoxicosis, before the axis recovers
        from suppression
Drugs
    Dopamine
    Glucocorticoids
Laboratory error
Secondary (pituitary) and tertiary (hypothalamic) hypothy-
        roidism (see 4-E)
Severe nonthyroidal illness

References

1. Ross DS: Subclinical Hypothyroidism, pp. 1010–1011.
   See Bibliography, 4.
2. Ross DS: Subclinical Thyrotoxicosis, pp. 1016–1017. See
   Bibliography, 4.

4-H. Radioactive Iodine Uptake

Factors Causing Increased Uptake
Reflecting increased hormone synthesis
    Excessive hormone losses
        Chronic diarrhea states
        Nephrosis
        Soybean ingestion
    Hyperthyroidism (see 4-D)
    Response to glandular hormone depletion
        Rebound after suppression of TSH
        Recovery phase of silent, subacute, or other transient
            destructive thyroiditis
        Rebound phase after withdrawal of iodide or other
            antithyroid drugs (if TSH is elevated)
Not reflecting increased hormone synthesis
    Iodide deficiency
        Dietary
        Excessive loss
            Dehalogenase defect
            Pregnancy
        Hashimoto's thyroiditis (if TSH is elevated)
        Inherited disorders of thyroid hormone synthesis
            (except for iodide trapping defects)
        Lithium administration

Factors Causing Decreased Uptake

Reflecting decreased hormone synthesis
- Primary hypofunction
  - Drugs (other than those containing iodide)
    - Major effect
      - Glucocorticoids (in large doses, acutely)
      - Paraaminobenzoic acid
      - Perchlorate
      - Salicylates (>5 g/day)
      - Sulfonamides
      - Thiocyanate
      - Thioamides
        - Carbimazole
        - Methimazole
        - Propylthiouracil
    - Minor effect
      - Aminoglutethimide
      - Phenylbutazone
      - Resorcinol (topical)
      - Sulfonylureas
  - Secondary (pituitary) or tertiary (hypothalamic) hypothyroidism
  - Some hormone biosynthetic defects (especially defects in iodide trapping)
  - Status post thyroidectomy, radioiodine, or external radiotherapy to the head/neck
  - Hashimoto's thyroiditis (end stage)
  - Transient thyroiditis (active phase)
    - Postpartum thyroiditis
    - Silent (painless) thyroiditis
    - Subacute (DeQuervain's, granulomatous) thyroiditis
- Secondary hypofunction
  - Exogenous thyroid hormone
Not reflecting decreased hormone synthesis
- Certain types of thyrotoxicosis
  - (see 4-D)
  - Rapid hormone release owing to very severe hyperthyroidism (rare)
- Increased nonradioactive iodide exposure
  - Cardiac or renal failure with iodide retention
  - Increased dietary iodide
  - Pharmacologic iodide exposure
    - Amiodarone
    - Other iodine-containing drugs
    - Iodide-containing x-ray contrast agents

References
1. Larsen PR, Davies TF, Hay ID: The Thyroid Gland, pp. 410–412. See Bibliography, 3.
2. Cavalieri RR, McDougall IR: In Vivo Isotopic Tests and Imaging, pp. 355–357. See Bibliography, 4.

4-I. Goiter/Neck Mass

Diffuse Goiter
Euthyroid or hypothyroid
   Cigarette smoking (thiocyanate)
   Increased intrinsic growth potential
   Exposure to thyroid growth factors
      Excess TSH
      Chemicals
         Cobalt
         Flavonoids (polyphenols)
         Organochlorines
            Polychlorinated and polybrominated biphenyls
            Polycyclic aromatic hydrocarbons
            Phthalate esters and metabolites
            Polyhydroxyphenols and phenol derivatives
               2,4-Dinitrophenol
               Resorcinol (topical)
            Pyridines
            Sulfurated organic compounds
               Isothiocyanate
               Thiocyanate
      Defects in thyroid hormone synthesis
      Drugs
         Amiodarone
         Aniline derivatives
            Amphenone B
            Aminoglutethimide
            p-Aminosalicylic acid
            Phenylbutazone
         Antithyroid drugs
            Carbimazole
            Methimazole
            Propylthiouracil
         Dimercaprol (British antilewisite)
         Ethionamide
         Iodide excess

Iopanoic acid
Ipodate
Lithium carbonate
Nicardipine
Paraaminobenzoic acid
Perchlorate
Tumor necrosis factor-α
Generalized resistance to thyroid hormone
Ingestion of goitrogens
Brassica genus (broccoli, brussels sprouts, cabbage, cauliflower, kale, rape, rutabagas, swedes, turnips)
Cyanaglucosides (bamboo shoots, cassava, lima beans, maize, sweet potatoes)
Kelp
Soybean milk/soybean flour
Iodide deficiency
Neonatal
Maternal antithyroid drug therapy
Maternal iodine therapy
Protein calorie malnutrition
Selenium deficiency (usually with concomitant iodine deficiency)
Insulin-like growth factor-I
Pregnancy
Thyroid growth immunoglobulins
Infiltration
Amyloidosis
Thyroiditis
Acute (suppurative) thyroiditis
Hashimoto's thyroiditis
Silent (painless) thyroiditis
Riedel's thyroiditis
Subacute (DeQuervain's, granulomatous) thyroiditis
Sarcoidosis
Hyperthyroid
Excessive stimulation by human chorionic gonadotropin
Gestational thyrotoxicosis (with hyperemesis)
Tumors
Choriocarcinoma
Embryonal cell carcinoma of the testis
Hydatidiform mole
Graves' disease
Hashitoxicosis
Inappropriate TSH secretion
Selective pituitary resistance to thyroid hormone

TSH-secreting pituitary tumor
Neonatal (mother with Graves' disease)
Silent (painless) thyroiditis
Subacute thyroiditis

Multinodular Goiter
Multiple adenomas
Nontoxic nodular goiter (same causes as euthyroid or
      hypothyroid; see 4-I)
Toxic multinodular goiter

Nongoiter Neck Masses
Branchial cleft cyst
Cystic hygroma
Thyroglossal duct cyst

References

1. Davis PJ, Davis FB: Nontoxic Goiter, pp. 338–341. See
Bibliography, 2.
2. Burrow GN: The Thyroid: Nodules and Neoplasia, pp.
521–529. See Bibliography, 6.
3. Barsano CP: Other Forms of Primary Hypothyroidism, pp.
768–773. See Bibliography, 4.

4-J. Solitary Thyroid Nodule

Thyroid Lesions
Adenoma (benign)
    Atypical
    Embryonal (trabecular)
    Fetal
    Hamartomatous adiposity
    Hürthle cell
    Microfollicular
    Papillary cystadenoma
    Simple
    Signet ring adenomas
Colloid nodule (macrofollicular adenoma)
Ectopic normal or tumoral tissue within the thyroid
    Parathyroid
    Thymic
Focal or asymmetric thyroiditis
    Acute (suppurative) thyroiditis

Pneumocystis carinii infection (in AIDS)
Hashimoto's thyroiditis
Riedel's struma
Subacute (DeQuervain's, granulomatous) thyroiditis
Malignancy
Anaplastic carcinoma
Carcinosarcoma
Follicular carcinoma
Lymphoma
Malignant form of histiocytosis X
Malignant hemangioendothelioma
Mixed papillary-follicular carcinoma
Medullary carcinoma
Metastases to the thyroid
Papillary carcinoma
Paraganglioma
Sarcoma, angiosarcoma, fibrosarcoma
Squamous cell carcinoma
Miscellaneous
Agenesis of one lobe
Asymmetric multinodular goiter
Compensatory hyperplasia after hemithyroidectomy
Focal granulomatous disease (e.g., sarcoidosis)
Hematoma
Simple cyst

Nonthyroid Lesions
Carotid aneurysm
Cystic hygroma
Dermoid
Fibrosis (including postradiation)
Hemangioma
Laryngocele/bronchocele
Lipoma
Lymph node
Parathyroid adenoma
Parathyroid cyst
Teratoma
Thyroglossal duct cyst

References
1. Wartofsky L, Ahmann AJ: The Thyroid Nodule, pp.
   345–347. See Bibliography, 1.
2. Mazzaferri EL: Management of a Solitary Thyroid Nodule.
   N Engl J Med 328:553–559, 1993.

4-K. Hypercortisolism

Acute or chronic physical illness
Alcoholism
Depression
Elevated levels of cortisol-binding globulin
    Congenital
    Estrogens
    Pregnancy
Pulsatile cortisol secretion (normal)
Cushing's syndrome
    ACTH-dependent Cushing's syndrome
        Pituitary tumor secreting ACTH
            Ectopic
            Intrasellar
        Ectopic ACTH production
            Appendicular carcinoma
            Carcinoids
                Bronchial carcinoid
                Carcinoids of the gut
                Oncocytic carcinoid of the kidney
                Ovarian carcinoid
                Pancreatic carcinoid
                Thymic carcinoid
            Colonic carcinoma
            Cystadenoma of the pancreas
            Epithelial carcinoma of the thymus
            Esophageal carcinoma
            Gastric carcinoma
            Ileal carcinoma
            Medullary carcinoma of the thyroid
            Melanoma
            Oat cell carcinoma of the lung
            Ovarian tumors
            Pancreatic islet cell carcinoma
            Paraganglioma
            Pheochromocytoma
            Prostatic carcinoma
            Squamous cell carcinomas
                Cervix
                Larynx
                Lung
        Ectopic corticotropin-releasing hormone–secreting tumor
            Bronchial carcinoid
            Gangliocytoma

Medullary carcinoma of the thyroid
Oat cell carcinoma of the lung
Prostatic carcinoma
Pheochromocytoma
ACTH-independent Cushing's syndrome
Factitious (surreptitious ingestion of glucocorticoids)
Iatrogenic (glucocorticoid therapy)
Primary adrenal tumor
Adenoma
Carcinoma
Adrenal hyperplasias causing Cushing's syndrome
Bilateral macronodular hyperplasia
ACTH-dependent
ACTH-independent
Bilateral micronodular dysplasia
With atrophy of intervening non-nodular cortex
Primary pigmented nodular adrenal disease
(autosomal dominant)
Sporadic
With hyperplasia of intervening non-nodular cortex
Gastrointestinal peptide-dependent adrenocortical
hyperplasia
Nodular adrenal hyperplasia secondary to abnormal
production of 21-deoxycortisol
Nodular adrenal hyperplasia secondary to abnormal
expression of beta adrenergic receptors on
adrenocortical cells

References

1. Schteingart GE: Cushing Syndrome, pp. 667–669. See
   Bibliography, 2.
2. Orth DN, Kovacs WJ: The Adrenal Cortex, pp. 569–595.
   See Bibliography, 3.
3. Kannan CR: The Adrenal Cortex, pp. 138–140. See
   Bibliography, 7.

4-L. Adrenal Insufficiency

Primary
Autoimmune/idiopathic
Congenital/genetic
Adrenal aplasia or hypoplasia
Adrenoleukodystrophy/adrenomyelodystrophy

Congenital adrenal hyperplasia
Hereditary unresponsiveness to ACTH (familial glucocorti-
coid deficiency)
Drugs
Inhibition of cortisol biosynthesis
Aminoglutethimide
Metyrapone
o, p-Dichlorodiphenyldichloroethane (Mitotane)
Drugs that cause adrenal insufficiency in patients with
limited pituitary or adrenal reserve
Etomidate
Ketoconazole
Spironolactone
Suramin
Trilostane
Acceleration of cortisol metabolism (usually causing adrenal
insufficiency only in patients with limited pituitary or
adrenal reserve, or patients on replacement gluco-
corticoid therapy)
Barbiturates
Phenytoin
Rifampin
Iatrogenic
Irradiation
Bilateral adrenalectomy
Infectious
AIDS
Cryptococcus
Cytomegalovirus
Lymphoma
Metastatic Kaposi's sarcoma
Mycobacterium avium complex
Toxoplasmosis
Tuberculosis
Fungal
Blastomycosis
Coccidioidomycosis
Cryptococcosis
Histoplasmosis
Moniliasis
Paracoccidioidomycosis
Torulopsosis
Syphilis
Tuberculosis
Infiltrative
Amyloidosis

    Hemochromatosis
    Sarcoidosis
Neoplastic
    Leukemic infiltration
    Lymphoma
    Metastatic cancer
Vascular
    Bilateral adrenal hemorrhage and/or infarction
        Anticoagulants
        Antiphospholipid syndrome
        Arteritis
        Coagulopathy
        Emboli
        Hypotension
        Interleukin-2 therapy
        Neonatal
        Postadrenal venography
        Pregnancy
        Sepsis
            Waterhouse-Friderichsen syndrome
        Surgery
        Thrombosis
        Trauma

Secondary (Pituitary) or Tertiary (Hypothalamic)*
    After removal of cortisol-secreting adrenal tumor
    After withdrawal of drugs that suppress ACTH
        ACTH
        Glucocorticoids
        Megestrol acetate

References

1. Orth DN, Kovacs WJ: The Adrenal Cortex, pp. 553–558. See Bibliography, 3.
2. Oelkers W: Adrenal Insufficiency. *N Engl J Med* 335:1206–1212, 1996.

*See 4-S.

4-M. Impotence

Drug-induced
    Antiadrenergic
        Benzhexol

Benztropine
Bethanidine
Debrisoquin
Guanethidine
Phenoxybenzamine
Phentolamine
Prazosin
Propranolol
Thioridazine
Antiandrogen
Cimetidine
Cyproterone acetate
Estrogens
Finasteride
Flutamide
Ketoconazole
Progestins
Ranitidine
Spironolactone
Anticholinergic
Atropine
Disopyramide
Ganglionic blocking agents
Tricyclic antidepressants
Central nervous system depressants
Alpha-methyldopa
Barbiturates
Benzodiazepines
Butyrophenones
Carbamazepine
Clonidine
Ethanol
Fluoxetine
Heroin
Methadone
Morphine
Phenothiazines
Phenytoin
Primidone
Reserpine
Other drugs
Amphetamines
Cocaine
Marijuana
Monoamine oxidase inhibitors
Thiazides

Endocrine
  Cushing's syndrome (see 4-K)
  Diabetes mellitus
  Feminizing adrenal or testicular tumors
  Hyperprolactinemia (see 4-R)
  Hypogonadism (see 4-N)
  Hypopituitarism (see 4-S)
  Hypothyroidism (see 4-E)
  Thyrotoxicosis (see 4-D)
Endurance factors
  Anemia
  Congestive heart failure
  Hepatic failure
  Postmyocardial infarction
  Pulmonary insufficiency
  Sleep disorders
  Systemic illnesses
  Uremia
Genitourinary
  Cystitis
  Genital malignancy
  Hydrocele
  Hypospadias
  Micropenis and other congenital deformities
  Pelvic fracture
  Penectomy
  Penile trauma
  Peyronie disease
  Phimosis
  Prostate irradiation
  Prostatitis
  Ruptured urethra
  Scleroderma
  Seminal vesiculitis
  Urethral stricture
  Urethritis
Neurologic
  Amyotrophic lateral sclerosis
  Arachnoiditis
  Autonomic neuropathy
  Bicycle rider's palsy
  Friedreich's ataxia
  Herniated disc
  Hypothalamic disease
  Multiple sclerosis
  Neurosyphilis (general paresis, tabes dorsalis)

Parkinsonism
Peripheral neuropathy
Pernicious anemia (subacute combined degeneration)
Shy-Drager syndrome
Spina bifida
Spinal cord syrinx
Spinal cord transection/injury
Spinal cord tumor
Temporal lobe disorders
Transverse myelitis
Psychogenic
Surgical
   Abdominal perineal resection
   Aortoiliac surgery
   External sphincterotomy
   Pelvic or retroperitoneal lymphadenectomy
   Perineal prostatectomy
   Perineal prostatic biopsy
   Rectosigmoid surgery
   Sympathectomy
   Vascular surgery (abdominal aortic aneurysm repair)
Vascular
   Aneurysm
   Aortoiliac arteriosclerosis
   Arterial dysplasia
   Arteritis
   Embolism
   Hypertension
   Leriche syndrome
   Priapism
   Thrombosis

References

1. Cunningham GR, Hershkowitz M: Impotence, pp. 1091–1096. See Bibliography, 2.
2. Korenman SG: Sexual Function and Dysfunction, p. 929. See Bibliography, 3.

4-N. Male Hypogonadism

Primary
Acquired
   Adult seminiferous tubule failure

Amyloidosis
Autoimmune destruction
Cryptorchidism
Drugs
    Chemotherapy
    Ethanol
    Ketoconazole
    Marijuana
    Spironolactone
Granulomatous disease
    Leprosy
Leukemia
Viral orchitis
    Mumps
Polyarteritis nodosa
Radiation
Surgery (castration)
Trauma
Developmental
  Congenital anorchia
  Decreased responsiveness to testosterone (male pseudo-
      hermaphroditism)
    Reifenstein's syndrome
    5α-Reductase deficiency
  Defective testosterone biosynthesis
  Functional prepubertal castrate (vanishing testes
      syndrome)
  Klinefelter's syndrome
  Luteinizing hormone (LH) resistant testes
  Myotonic dystrophy
  Persistent müllerian duct syndrome
  Sertoli-cell only syndrome
  Ullrich-Noonan syndrome (male Turner syndrome)
  XY/XO mixed gonadal dysgenesis
  XX male
  XYY syndrome

Secondary (Pituitary) or Tertiary (Hypothalamic)
Hypopituitarism (see 4-S)
Congenital adrenal hyperplasia
Constitutional delay of puberty
Cushing's syndrome (see 4-K)
Estrogen-secreting tumors
Exposure to estrogen in embalming compounds
Fröhlich's syndrome

Hyperprolactinemia (see 4-R)
Hypopituitarism (see 4-S)
Idiopathic hypogonadotropic hypogonadism (may be adult
    onset)
Isolated gonadotropin deficiency
    Hypogonadotropic eunuchoidism
        Complete (Kallman's syndrome)
        Partial
            Inherited immunologically active, biologically inac-
                tive LH
            Predominant LH deficiency, "fertile eunuch" syndrome
        Variant form (isolated follicle-stimulating hormone defi-
            ciency)
    Specific genetic syndromes
        Bardet-Biedl syndrome
        Börjeson-Forssman-Lehman syndrome
        Central nervous system (CNS) anomalies, genital
            hypoplasia, and ear anomalies and/or deafness
            (CHARGE) syndrome
        Laurence-Moon syndrome
        Lowe's syndrome
        Martsolf syndrome
        Möbius syndrome
        Multiple lentigines (leopard syndrome)
        Prader-Labhart-Willi syndrome
        Rothmund-Thomson syndrome
        Rud's syndrome
        Steroid sulfatase deficiency
Morbid obesity
Pituitary dwarfism
Severe illness (acute or chronic)
Withdrawal of androgen therapy (temporary)

Combined Primary and Secondary
Aging
Cirrhosis
Sickle cell disease

References
1. Plymate SR: Male Hypogonadism, pp. 1057–1079. See
   Bibliography, 2.
2. Santen RJ: The Testis, pp. 916–935. See Bibliography, 6.

4-O. Gynecomastia

Acromegaly
Chest wall trauma (including hip spica cast)
Drugs
    Amiodarone
    Amphetamines
    Androgens (aromatizable)
        Testosterone enanthate
        Testosterone propionate
    Angiotensin-converting enzyme inhibitors
    Antineoplastics (especially alkylating agents and cisplatin)
    Auranofin
    Busulfan
    Calcium channel blockers
    Cimetidine
    Clomiphene
    Cyproterone
    D-penicillamine
    Diazepam
    Diethylpropion
    Digitalis preparations
    Estrogens, phytoestrogens
    Ethionamide
    Etomidate
    Etretinate
    Finasteride
    Flutamide
    Gonadotropins
    Haloperidol
    Heroin
    Isoniazid
    Ketoconazole
    Marijuana
    Methyldopa
    Metronidazole
    Omeprazole
    Phenothiazines
    Phenytoin
    Progestogens
    Ranitidine
    Reserpine
    Spironolactone
    Sulindac
    Theophylline

Tricyclic antidepressants
Hyperprolactinemia (see 4-R)
Idiopathic gynecomastia
   Increased estrogen production
   Increased availability of estrogen precursors
      Congenital adrenal hyperplasia
         21-Hydroxylase deficiency
         11-Hydroxylase deficiency
      Liver disease (especially cirrhosis)
      Thyrotoxicosis
   Increased peripheral aromatase activity
      Hereditary
      Neoplasia
         Fibrolamellar hepatocellular carcinoma
         Testicular carcinomas
      Obesity
   True hermaphroditism
Male hypogonadism (see 4-N)
Neoplasms
   Secreting estrogens or estrogenic precursors
      Feminizing adrenal tumors
      Testicular tumors (especially Leydig cell tumors, Sertoli
         cell tumors, choriocarcinomas, and germinal
         epithelial tumors)
   Secreting gonadotropins
      Gonadotropin-secreting pituitary adenomas
   Secreting HCG
      Nontesticular tumors
         Gynecomastia reported with elevated HCG
            Adenocarcinoma of the stomach
            Carcinoma of the lung (especially bronchogenic
               carcinoma)
            Carcinoma of the pancreas
            Hepatoma, hepatoblastoma
            Renal cell carcinoma
            Undifferentiated mediastinal carcinoma
         Detectable HCG reported without gynecomastia (yet)
            Biliary tract
            Breast
            Colon/rectal
            Esophagus
            Insulinoma
            Leukemia
            Liver sarcoma
            Lymphoma
            Medullary carcinoma of the thyroid

Melanoma
Multiple myeloma
Ovarian
Pheochromocytoma
Sarcomas
Small intestine
Testicular tumors
Germ cell tumors of the testis (embryonal carci-
nomas, choriocarcinomas, teratomas, rarely
seminomas)
Secreting prolactin
Pituitary prolactinomas
Persistent pubertal macromastia
Physiologic
Normal physical finding
Neonatal
Pubertal
Senescent
Pseudogynecomastia
Obesity
Benign or malignant breast tumor
Psychological stress
Spinal cord injury
Systemic diseases (especially recovery from chronic disease)
HIV infection
Poorly controlled diabetes mellitus
Pulmonary tuberculosis
Refeeding gynecomastia (after starvation)
Uremia and dialysis

References

1. Glass AR: Gynecomastia, p. 1123. See Bibliography, 2.
2. Braunstein GD: Gynecomastia. *N Engl J Med*
   328:490–495, 1993.

4-P. Amenorrhea

Hypothalamic and Pituitary Causes

Androgen excess (see 9-D)
Chorionic gonadotropin-secreting tumors
Chronic debilitating diseases (e.g., liver disease, uremia,
regional ileitis)

Congenital hypothalamic hypogonadism
    Idiopathic
    With anosmia or hyposmia (Kallman's syndrome)
Cushing's syndrome
Defects in gonadotropin synthesis
Estrogen-secreting ovarian or adrenal tumors
Gonadotropin-secreting pituitary tumors
Hypopituitarism (see 4-S)
Hypothalamic-pituitary dysfunction due to extrinsic factors
    Anovulation
        Hypothyroidism
        Obesity
        Perimenopause
    Hyperprolactinemia (see 4-R)
    Lactation
    Nutritional
        Acute weight loss
        Malnutrition (including anorexia nervosa)
        Underweight
    Post-pill amenorrhea
    Pregnancy
    Pseudocyesis
    Strenuous exercise
    Stress
    Thyrotoxicosis
    Idiopathic delayed puberty
    Secretion of biologically inactive gonadotropin

Ovarian Causes

    Acquired (premature ovarian failure)
        Autoimmune
        Chemotherapy
        Idiopathic (premature menopause)
        Myotonic dystrophy
        Postinfection
            Mumps oophoritis
            Severe pelvic inflammatory disease
        Radiation
        Surgical castration
        Trauma
    Congenital
        Congenital thymic aplasia
        Galactosemia
        Gonadal agenesis
        Gonadal dysgenesis (including Turner's syndrome)

Ovarian enzymatic deficiency
   17α-Hydroxylase deficiency
   17,20-Lyase deficiency
Resistant ovary syndrome (Savage syndrome)
Sex chromosome mosaicism
Trisomy X
True hermaphroditism
XY gonadal dysgenesis
Menopause

Uterine and Outflow Tract Abnormalities

Female pseudohermaphroditism
   Congenital adrenal hyperplasia
   Exposure to maternal androgens *in utero*
Hysterectomy
Male pseudohermaphroditism
   5α-Reductase deficiency
   Complete and incomplete androgen insensitivity
   Enzymatic defects in testosterone biosynthesis
Müllerian agenesis
Müllerian anomalies
   Absence or anomalies of vagina, cervix, endometrium,
      or endometrial cavity
   Imperforate hymen
   Labial agglutination or fusion
Trauma (including surgical)
   Cervical stenosis
   Sclerosis of the uterine cavity (Asherman's syndrome)
      Abortion
      After uterine surgery (caesarian section, metro-
         plasty, myomectomy)
      Repeated or overzealous uterine curettage
      Severe, generalized pelvic infections
      Tuberculous endometritis
      Uterine schistosomiasis
   Vaginal stenosis

References

1. Speroff L, Glass RH, Kase NG: Amenorrhea. pp. 418–445.
   See Bibliography, 8.
2. McIver B, Romanski SA, Nippoldt TB: Evaluation and
   Management of Amenorrhea. *Mayo Clin Proc*
   72:1161–1169, 1997.

4-Q. Galactorrhea/Nipple Discharge

Galactorrhea
    Hyperprolactinemia (see 4-R)
    Normoprolactinemic galactorrhea
        Idiopathic galactorrhea with menses
        Post–oral contraceptive galactorrhea
Pseudogalactorrhea
    Intramammary lesions
        Benign
            Fibrocystic disease
            Intraductal papilloma
        Malignant neoplasm

References
1. Goldenberg IS: Nipple Discharge. *Postgrad Med* 70:116–117, 1981.
2. Blackwell RE: Pathophysiology of the Breast, pp. 974–975. See Bibliography, 2.

4-R. Hyperprolactinemia

Addison's disease
Adrenal carcinoma
Adrenal hyperplasia
Antiprolactin autoantibodies
Chronic renal failure
Cirrhosis
Diseases affecting the hypothalamus and/or pituitary stalk
    Aneurysms
    Basilar meningitis
    Empty sella syndrome
    Encephalitis/postencephalitis
    Giant cell arteritis
    Histiocytosis X
    Hydrocephalus
    Hypothalamic tumors, primary or metastatic (including craniopharyngiomas, dysgerminomas, gliomas, hamartomas, lymphomas, meningiomas, and pinealomas)
    Neuraxis irradiation

Pituitary stalk section (including pituitary tumors com-
    pressing the stalk)
Pseudotumor cerebri
Postpneumoencephalogram
Rathke's pouch cyst
Sarcoidosis
Trauma
Tuberculosis
Other destructive lesions of the hypothalamus
    (see 4-Q)
Drugs
Alpha-methyldopa
Alpha-methyl-para tyrosine
Amphetamines
Androgens
Antidepressants
    Dibenzoxazepine antidepressants (e.g., amoxapine)
    Tricyclic antidepressants
Antihistaminics (H1 and H2)
    Cimetidine
    Cyproheptadine
    Meclizine
    Tripelennamine
Benzodiazepines
Calcium channel blockers
Cocaine
Cyproterone acetate
Domperidone
Estrogens
Isoniazid
Medroxalol
Monoamine oxidase inhibitors
Meprobamate
Neuroleptics
    Azophenothiazines
    Benzisoxazoles
    Butyrophenones
    Dibenzooxazepines
    Dibenzothiazepines
    Dihydroindolones
    Phenothiazines
    Thioxanthenes
Opiates
Reserpine
Substituted benzamides
    Brompride

      Clebopride
      Cisapride (rare)
      Metoclopramide
      Sulpiride
    Tetrabenazine
    Thyrotropin-releasing hormone
Hypoglycemia
Idiopathic hyperprolactinemia
Macroprolactinemia
Neural stimulation
    Due to disorders of the chest wall and thorax
      Atopic dermatitis
      Bronchiectasis/chronic bronchitis
      Bronchogenic tumors
      Burns
      Chest wall lesions
      Chest wall scars
      Chest wall trauma
      Herpes zoster
      Mastectomy/mammoplasty
      Neoplasms of the chest wall
      Thoracotomy/thoracoplasty
      Tight garments
    Due to nipple stimulation
      Chronic inflammatory disease
      Mechanical stimulation of the nipples
    Due to psychogenic factors
      Pseudocyesis
      Posttrauma
      Stress
    Due to spinal cord disease
      Cervical ependymoma
      Cervical spinal cord lesions
      Extrinsic tumors
      Syringomyelia
      Tabes dorsalis
    Major surgery and anesthesia, especially oophorectomy
    Seizures
Physiologic causes of hyperprolactinemia
    Exercise
    Intercourse
    Newborn
    Postpartum
      Nonnursing (4 weeks)
      Suckling
    Pregnancy

    Sleep
Polycystic ovary syndrome
Primary hypothyroidism
Pseudohypoparathyroidism
Refeeding after starvation
Tumors secreting prolactin or placental lactogen
    Acromegaly
    Bronchogenic carcinoma
    Chorioepithelioma
    Hydatidiform mole
    Hypernephroma
    Prolactinoma
    Uterine leiomyoma

References
1. Katznelson L, Klibanski A: Prolactin and Its Disorders, pp. 141–143. See Bibliography, 2.
2. Reichlin S: Neuroendocrinology, p. 226. See Bibliography, 3.

4-S. Pituitary/Hypothalamic Insufficiency

Acquired during birth
    Asphyxia
    Breech delivery
    Intracranial hemorrhage or thrombosis
Acute intermittent porphyria
Chronic renal failure (TSH, gonadotropin deficiency)
Congenital
    Tumors
        Diencephalic syndrome
    Developmental
        Absence of anterior pituitary
        Anencephaly
        Basal encephalocele
        Cleft lip and palate
        Ectopic anterior pituitary
        Holoprosencephalic syndromes
        Optic nerve hypoplasia
        Single central incisor
    Mutations in the Pit-1 gene (TSH, growth hormone, pro-lactin deficiency)
Iatrogenic
    Radiation therapy

Therapy for head or neck tumor
To the pituitary
Vincristine
Idiopathic
Congenital
Familial
Sporadic
Necrotizing infundibulo-hypophysistis
Immunologic
Lymphocytic hypophysitis
Infectious
AIDS
Cytomegalovirus
Herpes simplex type 2 encephalitis
Brucellosis
Encephalitis
Fungal infections
Infected Rathke's cleft cyst
Malaria
Meningitis
Pyogenic abscess
Septic cavernous sinus
Syphilis
Tuberculosis
Infiltrative
Amyloidosis
Hemochromatosis
Histiocytosis X
Idiopathic granulomatous hypophysitis
Leukemia
Lipid storage diseases
Sarcoidosis
Tay-Sachs disease
Wegener's granulomatosis
Injury
Acute epidural and subdural hematoma
Basilar skull fracture
Subarachnoid hemorrhage
Post-traumatic chronic brain syndrome
Invasive
Aneurysm of the intracranial internal carotid artery
Arteriovenous anomalies
Craniopharyngioma
Empty sella syndrome
Metastases to the pituitary or hypothalamus (especially
        breast, lung, and melanoma)

Pituitary adenoma
Parasellar and hypothalamic tumors (e.g., glioma, menin-
            gioma, pinealoma, lymphoma)
Rathke's cleft cyst
Third ventricle cyst
Ischemic necrosis of the pituitary
    Arteriosclerosis
    Cavernous sinus thrombosis
    Collagen vascular disease
    Diabetes mellitus
    Eclampsia
    Pituitary apoplexy
    Sheehan's syndrome
    Sickle cell anemia (disease and trait)
    Temporal arteritis
Isolated
    Isolated ACTH deficiency
    Isolated gonadotropin deficiency
        Biologically inactive LH
        Kallman's syndrome
    Isolated growth hormone deficiency
        Biologically inactive/subactive growth hormone
        Deprivational dwarfism
        Growth hormone neurosecretory defect
    Isolated prolactin deficiency
    Isolated thyrotropin (TSH) deficiency
        Abnormal TSH β subunit secretion
    Isolated vasopressin deficiency

References
1. Dexter RN: Hypopituitarism, pp. 169–171. See
   Bibliography, 2.
2. Aron DC, Findling JW, Tyrrell JB: Hypothalamus and
   Pituitary, pp. 124–128. See Bibliography, 9.
3. Lamberts SWJ, deHerder WW, van der Lely AJ: Pituitary
   Insufficiency. *Lancet* 352:127–134, 1998.

4-T. Diabetes Insipidus

Nephrogenic
(See 6-B)

Central
Gestational diabetes insipidus (vasopressinase production)
Iatrogenic
   Surgery (hypophysectomy)
   Irradiation
Idiopathic
   Familial
      Isolated
         Autosomal dominant
         X-linked recessive
      Wolfram [DIDMOAD (diabetes insipidus, diabetes mel-
         litus, optic atrophy, deafness, atonia of bladder
         and ureters)] syndrome (autosomal recessive)
   Sporadic (one-third have circulating antibodies to vaso-
      pressin-producing cells)
Infection
   Actinomycosis
   AIDS
      CNS herpes
      CNS lymphoma
      Cytomegalovirus
      Toxoplasma gondii
   Basilar meningitis
   Blastomycosis
   Brain abscess
   Brucellosis
   Diphtheria
   Encephalitis
   Landry–Guillain-Barré syndrome
   Measles
   Mumps
   Scarlet fever
   Syphilis
   Tuberculosis
Infiltrative
   Amyloidosis
   Eosinophilic granuloma
   Histiocytosis X
   Sarcoidosis

Wegener's granulomatosis
Xanthoma disseminatum
Miscellaneous
    Circulating antibodies to vasopressin (secondary to
            Pitressin injection)
    Collagen vascular disease
    Empty sella syndrome (rarely)
    Fat embolus
    Hydrocephalus
    Lymphocytic hypophysitis
    Suprasellar and intrasellar cysts
Neoplasm
    Astrocytoma
    Craniopharyngioma
    Dysgerminoma
    Glioma
    Large pituitary adenoma
    Leukemia
    Lymphoma
    Meningioma
    Metastatic cancer (especially breast, lung, and melanoma)
    Pinealoma
Traumatic
    Birth trauma
    Head injury (basilar skull fracture)
    Post–cranial surgery
Vascular
    Aneurysm of the intracranial internal carotid artery
    Cardiopulmonary arrest
    Hypertensive encephalopathy
    Intraventricular hemorrhage
    Pituitary apoplexy
    Ruptured cerebral aneurysm
    Sheehan's syndrome
    Shock/hemorrhage
    Sickle cell crisis
    Thrombosis
    Thrombotic thrombocytopenic purpura
    Vasculitis

References
1. Moses AM, Streeten DHP: Disorders of the
   Neurohypophysis, pp. 2005–2006. See Bibliography, 1.
2. Baylis PH, Thompson CJ: Diabetes Insipidus and
   Hyperosmolar Syndromes, pp. 257–258. See
   Bibliography, 2.

4-U. Hyperlipidemia

Type I (Chylomicrons)
Primary
  Familial apolipoprotein C-II deficiency
  Familial lipoprotein lipase deficiency
  Inherited circulating lipoprotein inhibitor
Secondary
  Dysglobulinemias (lupus, lymphoma, myeloma,
      Waldenström's macroglobulinemia)
  Glycogen storage disease, type I
  High-dose glucocorticoids
  Severe untreated diabetes mellitus
  Tamoxifen therapy

Type IIA (Low-Density Lipoproteins) and IIB (Low-Density Lipoproteins + Very-Low-Density Lipoproteins)
Primary
  IIA only
    Familial defective apolipoprotein B100 [reduced affinity
        of low-density lipoproteins (LDL) for its receptor]
    Familial hypercholesterolemia
      Defective LDL receptors
      Deficiency of LDL receptors
      LDL internalization defect
      Polygenic hypercholesterolemia
  IIA and IIB
    Familial combined hyperlipidemia
Secondary
  IIA only
    Acute intermittent porphyria
    Anorexia nervosa
    Dysglobulinemias (lupus, lymphoma, myeloma,
        Waldenström's macroglobulinemia)
    Drugs
      Cyclosporine
      Glucocorticoids
      Progestogens
      Thiazides
    Excess dietary cholesterol
    Hypothyroidism
    Liver disease (abnormal levels of an abnormal lipopro-
        tein called lipoprotein X)
      Alpha₁-antitrypsin deficiency
      Biliary atresia

        Extrahepatic biliary obstruction
        Primary biliary cirrhosis
    Nephrotic syndrome
IIB only
    Diabetes mellitus (moderate)
    Familial hypercholesterolemia (rarely)
    Glucocorticoids
    Hypopituitarism (ateliotic dwarfism)
    Nephrotic syndrome
    Sitosterolemia
IIA and IIB
    Biliary obstruction
    Cushing's syndrome
    Diabetes mellitus (uncontrolled)
    Glucocorticoids (low dose)
    Hypothyroidism
    Nephrotic syndrome
    Pregnancy
    Thiazides
    Werner's syndrome

Type III (Intermediate-Density Lipoproteins)

Primary
    Familial dysbetalipoproteinemia
        Apolipoprotein E deficiency
        Apolipoprotein E_2 homozygotes
        Other apolipoprotein E variants
    Hepatic lipase deficiency
Secondary
    Beta blockers
    Diabetes mellitus
    Dysglobulinemias (lupus, lymphoma, myeloma,
        Waldenström's macroglobulinemia)
    Hypothyroidism (rarely)
    Obesity
    Thiazides
    Uremia

Type IV (Very-Low-Density Lipoproteins)

Primary
    Familial apolipoprotein C-II deficiency
    Familial combined hyperlipidemia
    Familial hypertriglyceridemia
    Familial lipoprotein lipase deficiency
    Lecithin-cholesterol acyltransferase (LCAT) deficiency
    Fish-eye disease (milder variant of LCAT deficiency)

Sporadic hypertriglyceridemia
Tangier disease
Secondary
Acromegaly
Acute hepatitis
Alcohol
Beta blockers
Cushing's syndrome
Diabetes mellitus (moderate)
Drugs
Beta blockers (but not those with intrinsic sympatho-
mimetic activity)
Bile acid–binding resins
Cimetidine
Estrogen or oral contraceptive therapy
Glucocorticoids
Isotretinoin
Thiazides
Dysglobulinemias (lupus, lymphoma, myeloma,
Waldenström's macroglobulinemia)
Glycogen storage disease, type I
Hypopituitarism (ateliotic dwarfism)
Ileal bypass surgery
Lipodystrophy (congenital or acquired)
Nephrotic syndrome
Obesity
Pancreatitis
Pregnancy
Sepsis
Stress
Uremia

Type V (Chylomicrons and Very-Low-Density Lipoproteins)
Primary
Familial apoprotein C-II deficiency
Familial combined hyperlipidemia (rare)
Familial hypertriglyceridemia (severe form)
Familial lipoprotein lipase deficiency
Secondary
Alcohol (rare)
Diabetes mellitus (moderate or severe)
Dysglobulinemias (lupus, lymphoma, myeloma,
Waldenström's macroglobulinemia)
Estrogen or oral contraceptive therapy (rare)
Glycogen storage disease, type I (rare)
High-dose glucocorticoids

Hypopituitarism (ateliotic dwarfism)
Hypothyroidism
Isotretinoin therapy
Lipodystrophy (congenital or acquired)
Nephrotic syndrome
Pregnancy
Uremia

Familial Lipoprotein (a) Excess

Low High-Density Lipoproteins
Primary
Apolipoprotein A$_1$ variants
Cerebrotendinous xanthomatosis
Familial apo A-I and apo C-III deficiency
Familial apo A-I, C-III and A-IV deficiency
Familial apo A-I Milano
Familial hypoalphalipoproteinemia
Fish-eye disease
High-density lipoproteins deficiency with planar xan-
        thomas
Lecithin-cholesterol acyltransferase deficiency
Tangier disease
Secondary
Cigarette smoking
Diabetes mellitus, type 2
Drugs
    Anabolic steroids
    Beta blockers
    Probucol
Low-fat diet
Malnutrition
Obesity
Physical inactivity
Puberty in boys

References
1. Ginsberg HN, Goldberg IJ: Disorders of Lipoprotein
   Metabolism, pp. 2142–2145. See Bibliography, 1.
2. Mahley RW, Weisgraber KH, Farese RV Jr: Disorders of
   Lipid Metabolism, pp. 1125–1138. See Bibliography, 3.

4-V. Hypoglycemia

Fasting Hypoglycemia
Overutilization of glucose
  Autoimmune
    Antiidiotypic antibodies to antiinsulin antibodies
    Antiinsulin antibodies
    Antiinsulin receptor antibodies (stimulating) (including
      type B extreme insulin resistance)
  Deficiency of enzymes of fat oxidation and ketogenesis
    Carnitine palmitoyltransferase deficiency (less common)
    Electron transport flavoprotein deficiency
    Electron transport flavoprotein dehydrogenase
      deficiency
    Hepatic hydroxymethyl glutaryl coenzyme A (HMG
      CoA) lyase deficiency
    Medium and long chain acyl-CoA dehydrogenase
      deficiency
    Short and long chain 3-OH acyl-CoA dehydrogenase
      deficiency
    Systemic carnitine deficiency
  Drug-induced overutilization (factitious or iatrogenic)
    Insulin
    Metformin accompanied by
      Deficient caloric intake
      Ethanol
      Strenuous exercise
      Other glucose-lowering agents (insulin, sulfonyl-
        ureas, probably repaglinide)
      Repaglinide
      Sulfonylureas
      Vacor (acutely)
  Extrapancreatic tumors
    Adrenocortical carcinomas
    Bulky mesenchymal tumors
      Fibrosarcomas
      Hemangiopericytomas
      Leiomyosarcomas
      Liposarcomas
      Lymphosarcomas
      Mesotheliomas
      Rhabdomyosarcomas
    Carcinoidlike tumors
    Gastrointestinal carcinomas
    Hepatomas

       Lymphomas/leukemias
       Other (teratoma, kidney, ovary)
    Insulin excess
       Discontinuation of total parenteral nutrition
          (transient)
       Erythroblastosis fetalis (transient)
       Infants of diabetic mothers (transient)
       Pancreatic beta cell disorders
          Adenomatosis
          Beckwith-Wiedemann syndrome
          Insulinoma
          Islet cell hyperplasia
          Leprechaunism
          Nesidioblastosis
    Prolonged exercise (less likely in trained athletes)
Underproduction of glucose
    Congestive heart failure
    Deficiencies of insulin counter-regulatory hormones
       Adrenal hyporesponsiveness of small for gestational
          age (SGA) babies
       Adrenal insufficiency
       Epinephrine deficiency (infants)
       Glucagon deficiency
       Growth hormone deficiency (children; adults after pro-
          longed fasting)
       Hypopituitarism (less common older than age 6 years)
          (see 4-S)
       Hypothyroidism (see 4-E)
       Uremia
    Drug- or toxin-induced hypoglycemia
       Angiotensin-converting enzyme inhibitors
       Acetaminophen
       Acetazolamide
       Aluminum hydroxide
       Anabolic steroids
       Azapropazone
       Beta blockers
       Buformin
       Carbutamide
       Chloramphenicol
       Chloroquine
       Chlorpromazine
       Cibenzoline
       Cimetidine
       Clofibrate (potentiates sulfonylureas)
       Coumarin derivatives

Cycloheptolamide
Diphenhydramine
Disopyramide
Doxepin
Ethylenediaminetetraacetic acid
Encainide
Ethanol (blood alcohol levels may not be elevated
    when patient is hypoglycemic)
Fenoterol
Guanethidine
Haloperidol
Hypoglycin (unripe ackee fruit ingestion, "Jamaican
    vomiting illness")
Imipramine
Indomethacin
Isoproterenol
Isoxsuprine
Lidocaine
Lithium
Mebanazine
Mebendazole
Mesoxylate
Methimazole (autoimmune insulin syndrome)
Monoamineoxidase inhibitors
Orphenadrine
Ouabain
Oxytetracycline
Paraaminobenzoic acid
Paraaminosalicylic acid
Penicillamine (autoimmune insulin syndrome)
Pentamidine
Perhexiline
Phenindione
Phenylbutazone
Potassium paraaminobenzoate
Probenecid
Propoxyphene (in chronic renal failure)
Pyritinol (autoimmune insulin syndrome)
Quinidine (in treatment of cerebral malaria)
Quinine (i.v., in treatment of cerebral malaria)
Ranitidine
Ritodrine
Salicylates (children, and topical application for psoria-
    sis in chronic renal failure patients)
Sulfadiazine
Sulfonamides

Terbutaline
Tris(hydroxymethyl)-aminomethane
Falciparum malaria (children)
Disorders of gluconeogenesis
  Genetic disorders of amino acid metabolism
    Disorders of branched-chain amino acid metabolism
      Glutaric aciduria (type II)
      Maple syrup urine disease
    Organic acidemias
      Methylmalonic acidemias
      Propionic acidemia
  Fructose-1,6-bisphosphatase deficiency
  Phosphoenolpyruvate carboxykinase deficiency
  Pyruvate carboxykinase deficiency
Glycogen synthesis and breakdown, disorders of
  Glycogen storage diseases
    Type I
      Glucose-6-phosphatase deficiency
      Glucose-6-phosphate translocase deficiency
    Type III (debranching enzyme deficiency)
    Type VI
      Hepatic glycogen phosphorylase deficiency
      Hepatic glycogen phosphorylase kinase deficiency
  Glycogen synthase deficiency
Hepatic dysfunction (severe)
Hypothermia
Idiopathic hypoglycemia of infancy and childhood
Kidney transplantation, in children
Lactic acidosis
Removal of pheochromocytoma
Reye's syndrome
Sepsis
Substrate deficiency
  Ackee fruit ingestion
  Fasting hypoglycemia of pregnancy (late)
  Ketotic hypoglycemia of infancy
  Severe malnutrition (including anorexia nervosa and
    extreme food faddism)
Transient neonatal hypoglycemia (felt secondary to inade-
    quate substrate or enzyme function), especially
  Maternal toxemia
  Prematurity
  Respiratory distress
  Small for gestational age
  Smaller of twins

Type I glucose transporter defect, inherited (in children—
normal plasma glucose but low cerebrospinal
fluid glucose)

Uremia

*Reactive Hypoglycemia**

Induced by glucose
Alimentary
Gastrojejunostomy
Partial or total gastrectomy
Peptic ulcer disease
Pyloroplasty
Rapid gastric emptying
Thyrotoxicosis
Vagotomy
Early type 2 diabetes mellitus (uncommon)
Endocrine deficiencies
Adrenal insufficiency
Hypothyroidism
Functional/idiopathic/spontaneous reactive hypoglycemia
Insulinoma (occasionally)
Induced by other substrates
Fructose intolerance, hereditary
Galactosemia
Leucine-induced hypoglycemia

Factors Causing Increased Frequency of Hypoglycemia in Previously Compensated Diabetic Patients

Adrenal insufficiency
Antiinsulin antibodies (as a result of exposure to exogenous
insulin)
Autoimmune (see 4-V)
Decreased caloric intake
Development of hypoglycemic unawareness
Drugs and toxins (see 4-V)
Ethanol
Hypopituitarism (see 4-S)
Hypothyroidism (see 4-E)
Increased exercise
Renal failure
Weight loss

References
1. Service FJ: Hypoglycemic Disorders. *N Engl J Med* 332:1144–1152, 1995.
2. Foster DW, Rubenstein AH: Hypoglycemia, pp. 2082–2084. See Bibliography, 1.

*Twenty-five percent of asymptomatic controls have been reported to have symptomatic hypoglycemia during 5-hour oral glucose tolerance tests. Consider a diagnosis of "pseudohypoglycemia": postprandial adrenergic symptoms with concomitant normal plasma glucose levels.

4-W. Hyperglycemia

Inadequate dietary preparation for glucose tolerance test
Impaired glucose tolerance
Gestational diabetes
Type 1 diabetes (B-cell destruction, usually leading to absolute insulin deficiency)
    Idiopathic
    Immune-mediated
Type 2 diabetes (may range from predominantly insulin resistance with relative insulin deficiency to a predominantly secretory defect with insulin resistance)
Other specific types
Diseases of the exocrine pancreas
    Cystic fibrosis
    Fibrocalculous pancreatopathy
    Hemochromatosis
    Neoplasia
    Pancreatitis, acute, chronic or recurrent (usually with exocrine insufficiency)
    Trauma/pancreatectomy
Drug or toxin-induced
    ACTH
    α-Adrenergic agents
    Asparaginase
    Barium
    Benzodiazepines
    β-Adrenergic blockers
    Cadmium
    Calcium
    Calcium channel blockers
    Chlorpromazine
    Clonidine

Danazol
Dapsone
Dichlorodiphenyl-trichloroethane
Diazoxide
Estrogens, including oral contraceptives
Ethanol
Fluoride
Ganciclovir
Glucagon
Glucocorticoids
Growth hormone
Histaminergic blockers
Indomethacin
α-Interferon
Lithium
Mithramycin
Nicotinic acid
Octreotide
Opiates
Oxymetholone
Pentamidine (after initial hypoglycemia)
Phenothiazines
Phenytoin
Potassium
Prazosin
Protease inhibitors
    Didanosine
    Nelfinavir
Rifampin
Salicylates
Somatostatin
Sympathomimetic agents
Thiazides and (less-well substantiated) loop diuretics
Thyroid hormone
Trimethoprim-sulfamethoxazole
Vacor
Zinc
Endocrinopathies
    Increased counterregulatory hormones due to stress
        Hepatic insufficiency
        Infection
        Myocardial infarction
        Renal insufficiency
        Stroke
        Surgery
        Trauma

Disorders of increased counterregulatory hormone
    production
  Acromegaly
  Carcinoid syndrome
  Cushing's syndrome
  Glucagonoma
  Hyperaldosteronism (hypokalemia)
  Hyperprolactinemia
  Hyperthyroidism
  Pheochromocytoma
  Somatostatinoma
  VIPoma
Genetic defects in insulin action
  Leprechaunism
  Lipoatrophic diabetes
  Rabson-Mendenhall syndrome
  Type A insulin resistance
Genetic defects of B-cell function
  Chromosome 7, glucokinase (formerly MODY2)
  Chromosome 12, HNF-1α (formerly MODY3)
  Chromosome 20, HNF-α (formerly MODY1)
  Mitochondrial DNA
Infections
  Congenital rubella
  Cytomegalovirus
Uncommon forms of immune-mediated diabetes
  Antiinsulin receptor antibodies
  "Stiff-man" syndrome
Syndromes associated with increased risk of hyperglycemia
  Acute intermittent porphyria
  Alström's syndrome
  Ataxia telangiectasia
  Cockayne's syndrome
  Down's syndrome
  Friedreich's ataxia
  Glycogen storage disease, type I
  Hermann syndrome
  Huntington's chorea
  Isolated growth hormone deficiency
  Klinefelter's syndrome
  Laurence-Moon-Biedl syndrome
  Leprechaunism
  Lipodystrophic syndromes
  Machado disease
  Mutant insulins (e.g., insulin Chicago)
  Myotonic dystrophy

Panhypopituitary dwarfism
Prader-Willi syndrome
Turner's syndrome
Werner's syndrome
Wolfram (DIDMOAD) syndrome

Factors Causing Worsening of Previously Compensated Diabetes (see 3-I)

Decreased exercise
Drugs and toxins (see previous Drug or Toxin-Induced)
Endocrinopathies (see previous Endocrinopathies)
Increased caloric intake
Infection
Myocardial infarction
Pregnancy
Stroke
Surgery
Trauma
Weight gain

References

1. Expert Committee on the Diagnosis and Classification of Diabetes Mellitus: Report of the Expert Committee on the Diagnosis and Classification of Diabetes Mellitus. *Diabetes Care* 20(7):1183–1197, 1997.
2. Catanese VM, Kahn CR: Secondary Forms of Diabetes Mellitus, pp. 1220–1226. See Bibliography, 2.
3. Pandit MK, Burke JB, Gustafson AB, et al: Drug-Induced Disorders of Glucose Tolerance. *Ann Intern Med* 118:529–539, 1993.

Bibliography

1. Fauci AS, et al (eds): *Harrison's Principles of Internal Medicine*, 14/e. New York: McGraw-Hill, 1998.
2. Becker KL (ed): *Principles and Practice of Endocrinology and Metabolism*, 2/e. Philadelphia: JB Lippincott Co, 1995.
3. Wilson JD, Foster DW, Kronenberg HM, Larsen PR (eds): *Williams' Textbook of Endocrinology*, 9/e. Philadelphia: WB Saunders, 1998.
4. Braverman LE, Utiger RD (eds): *Werner and Ingbar's The Thyroid: A Fundamental and Clinical Text*, 7/e. Philadelphia: Lippincott–Raven, 1996.

5. Bennet JC, Plum F (eds): *Cecil Textbook of Medicine.* 20/e. Philadelphia: WB Saunders, 1996.
6. Felig P, Baxter JD, Frohman LA (eds): *Endocrinology and Metabolism,* 3/e. New York: McGraw-Hill, 1995.
7. Bagdade JD, et al. (eds): *Yearbook of Endocrinology 1996.* St. Louis: Mosby–Year Book, 1996.
8. Speroff L, Glass RH, Kase NG: *Clinical Gynecologic Endocrinology and Infertility,* 5/e. Baltimore: Williams & Wilkins, 1994.
9. Greenspan FS, Strewler GJ (eds): *Basic and Clinical Endocrinology,* 5/e. Stamford, CT: Appleton & Lange, 1997.

5
GASTROINTESTINAL AND HEPATIC SYSTEMS

5-A. Nausea and Vomiting*

Central Nervous System Disorders
Increased intracranial pressure
    Head trauma
    Central nervous system neoplasms
    Meningitis, encephalitis
    Hydrocephalus
    Pseudotumor
    Reye's syndrome
Vestibular or middle ear disease
    Motion sickness
    Ménière's disease
    Acoustic neuroma
    Labyrinthitis
    Ear infections
Eye disorders
    Glaucoma
    Refractive error
Vascular causes
    Migraine headache
    Migraine equivalent
Psychiatric causes
    Cyclical vomiting syndrome
    Psychogenic vomiting
    Self-induced (anorexia, bulimia)
    Concealed vomiting
    Erotic vomiting

Conditioned reflexes
Drug withdrawal
Rumination

Gastrointestinal Disorders

Mechanical intestinal obstruction (see 5-I)
Inflammatory/mass effect
    Gastroesophageal reflux disease
    Peptic ulcer disease
    Gastritis
    Bile reflux gastritis
    Crohn's disease
    Eosinophilic gastroenteritis
    Pancreatic pseudocyst
    Carcinoma/lymphoma of gastrointestinal tract or pancreaticobiliary system
    Abdominal carcinomatosis
    Graft-versus-host disease
    Duodenal hematoma
    Pneumatosis intestinalis
    Intestinal ischemia
    Prior gastric surgery
Visceral pain
    Severe pain of any cause
    Pancreatitis
    Cholecystitis
    Biliary stricture
    Choledocholithiasis
    Appendicitis
    Peritonitis
    Perforation
Functional intestinal obstruction
    Gastroparesis
        Diabetes
        Scleroderma
        Amyloidosis
        Metabolic
        Postoperative (postvagotomy)
        Postviral
        Idiopathic
    Pseudo-obstruction
        Chronic idiopathic intestinal pseudo-obstruction
        Colonic pseudo-obstruction (Ogilvie's syndrome)
    Adynamic ileus

Gastric motility disorders
Irritable bowel syndrome
Nonulcer dyspepsia

Pregnancy
Nausea and vomiting of pregnancy
Hyperemesis gravidarum
Acute fatty liver of pregnancy

Infections
Acute infections (especially children)
Systemic infections and sepsis
Food poisoning
Bacterial gastroenteritis
Helicobacter pylori infection
Hepatitis
Epidemic vomiting (Norwalk, Hawaii agent, etc.)
Viral gastroenteritis
Intestinal parasitic infestation
Gastric herpes, cytomegalovirus (CMV) (immunocompro-
        mised host)
Acquired immunodeficiency syndrome (AIDS)

Endocrine and Metabolic Disorders
Diabetic ketoacidosis
Metabolic acidosis
Uremia
Hypercalcemia
Hyponatremia
Hypothyroidism
Hyperthyroidism
Hyperparathyroidism
Adrenal insufficiency

Genitourinary Disorders
Pyelonephritis
Obstructive uropathy
Renal calculi
Salpingitis
Endometritis
Endometriosis

Drugs
Chemotherapeutic agents
Antiarrhythmics
Antibiotics
Anticholinergic drugs
Cardiac glycosides (digitalis)
Ergot alkaloids
Estrogens, oral contraceptives
Theophylline
Colchicine
Narcotics
Ipecac
Potassium chloride

Toxins
Alcohol
Carbon monoxide
Carbon tetrachloride
Heavy metals
Illicit drugs

Other
Acute myocardial infarction
Congestive heart failure
Radiation sickness
Radiation therapy

References
1. Ouyang A: Approach to the Patient with Nausea and Vomiting, pp. 647–659. See Bibliography, 5.
2. Lee M, Feldman M: Nausea and Vomiting, pp. 117–127. See Bibliography, 1.
3. Achord JL: Nausea and Vomiting, pp. 41–48. See Bibliography, 2.

*The causes of nausea and vomiting are innumerable; this list is not intended to include them all. The important categories of disorders with vomiting as a major symptom are listed, and several examples of each are given.

5-B. Dysphagia, Odynophagia

Oropharyngeal Dysphagia
Inflammation/infection
  Herpes stomatitis
  Monilial stomatitis
  Pharyngitis
  Vincent's angina
  Retropharyngeal abscess
  Peritonsillar abscess
  Caustic ingestion
  Mumps
  Stevens-Johnson syndrome
Structural abnormalities
  Intrinsic
    Postcricoid web
    Zenker's diverticulum
    Upper esophageal stricture
    Upper esophageal tumors
    Head and neck tumors
    Postsurgical change
    Postradiation change
    Foreign body
    Congenital anomalies
  Extrinsic
    Cervical osteophyte
    Thyromegaly
    Cricopharyngeal bar
    Cervical lymphadenopathy
    Vascular anomalies
Neurologic disorders
  Central nervous system disorders
  Cerebrovascular accident
  Parkinson's disease
  Brainstem tumors
  Alzheimer's disease
  Depression
  Tardive dyskinesia and dystonia
  Stiff-man syndrome
  Cerebral palsy
  Motor neuron disease (e.g., amyotrophic lateral
      sclerosis)
  Multiple sclerosis
  Poliomyelitis
  Huntington's chorea

Syringobulbia
Tabes dorsalis
Spinocerebellar degeneration
Cranial nerve diseases
Recurrent laryngeal nerve palsy
Cranial nerve injury
Rabies
Diphtheria
Peripheral neuropathies
Diabetic neuropathy
Lead poisoning
Neuromuscular diseases
Myasthenia gravis
Botulism
Skeletal muscle diseases
Muscular dystrophies
Oculopharyngeal dystrophy
Myotonic dystrophy
Polymyositis
Dermatomyositis
Connective tissue diseases
Scleroderma
Lupus erythematosus
Mixed connective tissue disease
Rheumatoid arthritis
Metabolic myopathies
Hyperthyroidism
Hypothyroidism
Amyloidosis
Other causes
Cricopharyngeal dysfunction
Xerostomia
Medication-induced
Sjögren's syndrome
Radiation-induced

Esophageal Dysphagia
Inflammation/infection
Reflux esophagitis
Bile reflux esophagitis
Radiation esophagitis
Caustic ingestion
Medication-induced esophagitis
Esophageal trauma
Esophageal infection

        CMV
        Herpes simplex virus (HSV)
        Idiopathic human immunodeficiency virus ulcers
        Esophageal moniliasis
    Esophageal Crohn's disease
    Eosinophilic esophagitis
    Esophageal sarcoidosis
    Graft-versus-host disease
    Behçet's syndrome
Structural abnormalities
    Intrinsic
        Esophageal stricture
        Esophageal carcinoma
        Carcinoma of the gastric cardia
        Esophageal benign tumor
        Esophageal web
        Esophageal ring (e.g., Schatzki's ring)
        Midesophageal diverticulum
        Epiphrenic diverticulum
        Esophageal pseudodiverticulosis
        Paraesophageal hernia
        Esophageal foreign body
    Extrinsic
        Vascular ring
        Cervical osteophyte
        Carcinoma of the lung
        Mediastinal lymphoma
        Mediastinal tuberculosis   .
        Pulmonary abscess
        Empyema
        Enlarged right atrium
        Pericardial effusion
        Enlarged aorta (dysphagia aortica)
        Anomalous right subclavian artery (dysphagia lusoria)
Motility disorders
    Primary
        Achalasia
        Nonspecific esophageal motility disorder
        Nutcracker esophagus
        Hypertensive lower esophageal sphincter
        Diffuse esophageal spasm
    Secondary
        Scleroderma and other connective tissue diseases
        Polymyositis
        Dermatomyositis
        Diabetes mellitus

Amyloidosis
Hyperthyroidism
Hypothyroidism
Chagas' disease
Pseudoachalasia
Chronic idiopathic intestinal pseudo-obstruction
Alcoholism
Paraneoplastic syndrome

References
1. See Bibliography, 6.
2. Richter JE: Dysphagia, Odynophagia, Heartburn, and Other Esophageal Symptoms, pp. 97–105. See Bibliography, 1.
3. Clouse RE, Diamant NE: Motor Physiology and Motor Disorders of the Esophagus, pp. 467–494. See Bibliography, 1.

5-C. Abdominal Pain*

Abdominal Disorders
Inflammatory disorders
Peritoneum
Peritonitis (chemical or bacterial; see 5-J)
Subdiaphragmatic abscess
Familial Mediterranean fever
Hollow viscera
Gastritis
Duodenitis
Peptic ulcer disease
Gastroenteritis
Cholecystitis
Bacterial cholangitis
Peptic ulcer disease
Intestinal perforation
Meckel's diverticulum
Appendicitis
Crohn's disease
Colitis (idiopathic and infectious)
Diverticulitis
Solid viscera
Pancreatitis (see 5-K)
Hepatitis (see 5-O)

Pyelonephritis
Abscess (especially hepatic, splenic, pancreatic, peri-
nephric, psoas)
Mesenteric lymphadenitis
Mechanical disorders
Hollow viscera
Intestinal obstruction
Intussusception
Volvulus
Biliary tract obstruction (stones, strictures)
Ureteral obstruction
Solid viscera
Acute capsular distention
Acute splenomegaly
Acute hepatomegaly (especially hepatitis, hepatic
congestion)
Nephrolithiasis
Abdominal wall
Abdominal wall contusion
Abdominal wall hematoma
Neoplasms
Pancreatic tumors
Gastric tumors
Hepatic tumors, primary or metastatic
Colonic tumors
Small intestinal tumors
Abdominal wall tumors
Vascular disorders
Intraabdominal bleeding
Ischemia
Mesenteric artery insufficiency or thrombosis
Mesenteric venous thrombosis
Budd-Chiari syndrome
Infarction (especially liver, spleen)
Omental ischemia
Abdominal aortic aneurysm
Functional disorders
Irritable bowel syndrome
Nonulcer dyspepsia
Sphincter of Oddi dysfunction
Functional constipation

Pelvic Disorders
Inflammatory disorders
Pelvic inflammatory disease
Tuboovarian disease

    Mittelschmerz
    Endometritis
    Endometriosis
    Salpingitis
    Fitz-Hugh–Curtis syndrome
    Cystitis
    Seminal vesiculitis
    Epididymitis
Mechanical disorders
    Ovarian cyst/torsion
    Ectopic pregnancy
    Distended bladder
    Omental torsion
Neoplasms
    Cervical tumors
    Ovarian tumors
    Uterine tumors
    Bladder tumors
    Prostate tumors

Extraabdominal Disorders
Thoracic
    Esophagitis
    Esophageal spasm
    Esophageal rupture (Boerhaave's syndrome)
    Myocardial infarction or ischemia
    Pericarditis
    Myocarditis
    Endocarditis
    Congestive heart failure
    Pneumonia
    Pulmonary embolism or infarction
    Pneumothorax
    Empyema
    Pleuritis
Neurologic
    Radiculitis
        Herpes zoster (shingles)
        Degenerative arthritis
        Herniated intervertebral disc
        Spinal or peripheral nerve tumors
    Causalgia
    Tabes dorsalis
    Abdominal epilepsy
Hematologic
    Leukemia

      Lymphoma
      Sickle cell anemia
      Hemolytic anemia
      Henoch-Schönlein purpura
Toxins
      Insect bite
      Snake bite
      Lead poisoning
Metabolic disorders
      Uremia
      Diabetes mellitus
      Diabetic ketoacidosis
      Acute adrenal insufficiency (Addison's disease)
      Porphyria
      Hypercalcemia
      Hyperparathyroidism
      Hyperlipidemia
      Hereditary angioneurotic edema
Psychiatric disorders
      Depression
      Anxiety disorders
      Schizophrenia
      Factitious abdominal pain
Other
      Acute glaucoma
      Narcotic withdrawal
      Heat stroke
      Unexplained intractable abdominal pain

References

1. Glasgow RE, Mulvihill SJ: Abdominal Pain, Including the Acute Abdomen, pp. 80–89. See Bibliography, 1.
2. Haubrich WS: Abdominal Pain, pp. 11–29. See Bibliography, 2.

*See also 5-D.

5-D. Characteristic Location of Abdominal Pain Associated with Various Diseases*

Diffuse
Gastroenteritis
Peritonitis

Pancreatitis
Leukemia
Sickle cell crisis
Early appendicitis (may be periumbilical)
Mesenteric adenitis
Mesenteric thrombosis
Abdominal aortic aneurysm
Intussusception
Colitis
Intestinal obstruction
Inflammatory bowel disease
Metabolic, toxic, bacterial causes

Epigastric
Reflux esophagitis
Peptic ulcer disease
Pancreatitis
Gastritis
Cholecystitis
Myocardial ischemia
Pericarditis
Abdominal wall hematoma

Right Upper Quadrant
Cholecystitis
Choledocholithiasis
Hepatitis
Hepatic metastases
Hepatic abscess
Hepatocellular carcinoma
Hepatomegaly resulting from congestive heart failure
Budd-Chiari syndrome (hepatic vein obstruction)
Peptic ulcer
Pancreatitis
Retrocecal appendicitis
Renal pain
Herpes zoster
Pulmonary infarction
Pleuritis

Left Upper Quadrant
Gastritis
Peptic ulcer disease
Pancreatitis
Splenomegaly or splenic rupture
Infarction, aneurysm

Renal pain
Herpes zoster
Myocardial ischemia
Pericarditis
Pneumonia
Empyema
Pulmonary infarction
Pleuritis

Right Lower Quadrant
Appendicitis
Intestinal obstruction
Crohn's disease
Diverticulitis
Cholecystitis
Perforated ulcer
Leaking aortic aneurysm
Abdominal wall hematoma
Ectopic pregnancy
Ovarian cyst or torsion
Salpingitis
Mittelschmerz
Endometriosis
Ureteral colic
Renal pain
Seminal vesiculitis
Psoas abscess

Left Lower Quadrant
Diverticulitis
Intestinal obstruction
Colon cancer
Appendicitis
Gastritis
Leaking aortic aneurysm
Inflammatory bowel disease
Abdominal wall hematoma
Splenomegaly
Ectopic pregnancy
Mittelschmerz
Ovarian cyst or torsion
Salpingitis
Endometriosis
Ureteral colic
Renal pain
Seminal vesiculitis

Psoas abscess
Irritable bowel syndrome

5-E. Constipation

Behavioral/Psychiatric Factors
Low-residue diet
Chronic laxative and/or enema abuse
Immobility
Reduced food intake
Repressed urge to defecate
Psychosis
Depression
Eating disorders
Obsessive/compulsive disorders

Functional Constipation
Simple (idiopathic) constipation
Irritable bowel syndrome
Slow transit
Outlet delay, anismus
Fecal impaction
Pseudo-obstruction

Gastrointestinal Disorders
Colonic extraluminal obstruction
  Intraabdominal or pelvic tumors
  Chronic volvulus
  Hernias
  Rectal prolapse
  Ascites
  Late pregnancy
  Adhesions
Colonic luminal obstruction
  Carcinoma of the colon or rectum
  Benign colonic tumors
  Recurrent diverticulitis
  Diverticular stricture

Colonic stricture
Chronic ulcerative colitis
Eosinophilic colitis
Chronic amebiasis
Lymphogranuloma venereum
Syphilis
Tuberculosis
Ischemic colitis
Endometriosis
Postsurgical abnormalities
Intussusception
Corrosive enemas
Anorectal disorders
Proctitis (especially ulcerative)
Hemorrhoids
Fissures and fistulas (e.g., Crohn's disease)
Perianal abscess
Rectal prolapse
Anterior mucosal prolapse
Anal atresia or malformation
Anal stenosis
Solitary rectal ulcer syndrome
Internal intussusception
Hereditary internal anal sphincter myopathy
Carcinoma of the rectum or anus
Ulcerative proctitis
Lymphogranuloma venereum
Postsurgical
Descending perineum syndrome
Rectocele

Endocrine/Metabolic Causes

Hypothyroidism
Hypercalcemia
Porphyria
Pheochromocytoma
Panhypopituitarism
Diabetes mellitus
Uremia
Hypokalemia
Heavy metal poisoning
Pregnancy
Glucagonoma
Pseudohypoparathyroidism

Neuromuscular Disorders
Parkinson's disease
Cerebrovascular accident
Brain tumors
Senile dementia
Multiple sclerosis
Tabes dorsalis
Spinal lesions
Aganglionic megacolon (Hirschsprung's disease)
Neurofibromatosis
Multiple endocrine neoplasia type 2b
Diabetic autonomic neuropathy
Chagas' disease
Familial visceral myopathy
Muscular dystrophies
Likongo's syndrome (hindgut dysgenesis)
Scleroderma
Amyloidosis
Hypoganglionosis and hyperganglionosis
Intestinal pseudoobstruction
Dermatomyositis

Drugs
Antacids
    Calcium carbonate
    Aluminum hydroxide
Opiates
Anticholinergics
Anticonvulsants
Tricyclic antidepressants
Ganglionic blockers
Phenothiazines
Diuretics
Ferrous sulfate
Antihypertensives
Barium sulfate
Bismuth compounds
Ion-exchange resins
Antispasmodics
Antidepressants
Antipsychotics
Calcium channel blockers
Calcium supplements
Sucralfate
Cholestyramine

Monoamine-oxidase (MAO) inhibitors
Analgesics
Vinca alkaloids

References:

1. Lennard-Jones JE: Constipation, pp. 174–197. See Bibliography, 1.
2. Koch TR: Constipation, pp. 102–112. See Bibliography, 2.

5-F. Diarrhea

Acute Diarrhea
Infections
    Viral gastroenteritis (adenovirus, Norwalk agent,
         rotavirus, etc.)
    Bacterial
        Invasive (e.g., *Shigella, Salmonella, Campylobacter,*
           Escherichia coli, Yersinia)
        Toxigenic (e.g., *Staphylococcus, E. coli, Clostridium dif-*
           ficile, Vibrio sp., toxic shock syndrome)
    Food poisoning
        Staphylococcus aureus
        Bacillus cereus
        C. perfringens
    Protozoal (e.g., amebiasis, giardiasis, cryptosporidium,
         Cyclospora)
    Fungal
    AIDS
        AIDS enteropathy
        Bacterial infections (see previous Bacterial listing)
        Cryptosporidium
        Microsporidium
        Amebiasis
        Giardiasis
        Isospora belli
        CMV
        HSV
        Adenovirus
        Mycobacterium avium complex
        Cryptococcus
        Histoplasma
        Candida

Stress-induced
Food allergy (rare)
Dietary indiscretion (e.g., prunes, unripe fruit, rhubarb,
        olestra)
Gastrointestinal disorders
   Partial bowel obstruction
   Fecal impaction
   Diverticulitis
   Appendicitis
   Ischemic bowel disease
   Initial attack of ulcerative colitis or Crohn's disease
Systemic/extraintestinal disorders
   Uremia
   Carcinoid syndrome
   Endocrine disorders
   Thyrotoxicosis
   Addisonian crisis
   Pelvic inflammation
Drugs/toxins (partial list)
   Laxatives (poorly absorbable sugars, fiber)
   Antibiotics
   Magnesium-containing antacids/products
   Colchicine
   Digitalis
   Iron
   Antihypertensives (methyldopa, hydralazine, and
        others)
   Quinidine
   Antidepressants (e.g., Prozac, Wellbutrin)
   Cisapride
   Valproic acid
   Antiretrovirals
   Protease inhibitors
   5-Aminosalicylic acid products
   Metformin
   Interferon products
   Immunosuppressives (cyclosporine, tacrolimus)
   Potassium preparations
   Nonsteroidal antiinflammatory drugs (NSAIDs)
   Lipid lowering agents
   Alcohol
   Heavy metals (especially arsenic, cadmium, mercury)
   Mushrooms
Acute exacerbation of chronic diarrhea

Chronic Diarrhea
Osmotic diarrhea
   Carbohydrate malabsorption
      Ingestion of poorly absorbable carbohydrates (sorbitol,
         mannitol fructose, lactulose, fiber)
      Congenital disaccharidase deficiencies
      Lactase deficiency
      Isomaltase-sucrase deficiency
      Trehalase deficiency
      Acquired disaccharidase deficiencies
         Nontropical sprue
         Tropical sprue
         Viral gastroenteritis
   Maldigestion syndromes (see 5-G)
   Malabsorption syndromes (see 5-G)
   Osmotic solutes
      Magnesium-containing laxatives
      Magnesium-containing antacids
      Magnesium-containing nutritional supplements
      Sodium citrate
      Sodium phosphate
      Sodium sulfate
      Polyethylene-glycol lavage solution
      Enteral feedings
   Reduced absorptive surface
      Intestinal resection
      Intestinal bypass
   Other osmotic causes
      Congenital chloridorrhea
      Postgastrectomy "dumping" syndrome
Secretory diarrhea
   Stimulant laxatives
      Bisacodyl
      Cascara
      Senna
      Ricinoleic acid
      Phenopthalein
      Docusate sodium
      Aloe
      Danthron
   Infections
      Enterotoxigenic bacteria (*E. coli*, cholera)
      Enteroviruses (Norwalk agent, rotavirus)
      Chronic infections (mycobacterial, fungal, parasitic)
      Bacterial overgrowth (intestinal stasis)
      AIDS (see previous Acute Diarrhea section)

Inflammation
   Crohn's disease
   Ulcerative colitis
   Lymphocytic colitis
   Collagenous colitis
   Celiac disease
Neoplasms
   Zollinger-Ellison syndrome (gastrinoma)
   Pancreatic cholera syndrome (VIPoma)
   Carcinoid syndrome
   Medullary carcinoma of the thyroid
   Glucagonoma
   Sympathetic tissue tumors (ganglioneuromas)
   Villous adenoma
   Carotid body tumor
   Pheochromocytoma
   Intestinal lymphoma [especially in human immunodefi-
      ciency virus (HIV) infection]
Other
   Fatty acid malabsorption
   Pancreatic insufficiency
   Bile acid malabsorption
   Postcholecystectomy bile acid–induced diarrhea
   Postvagotomy diarrhea
   Congenital absorptive defects
   Hyperthyroidism
   Collagen vascular disease
   Intestinal resection
   Hypoparathyroidism
   Addison's disease
   Food allergy
Exudative diarrhea
Infectious causes
   Bacterial/viral infections (see previous Acute Diarrhea
      section)
   Amebic colitis
   Parasitic infestation
   Pseudomembranous colitis
   Diverticulitis
Idiopathic and other colitides
   Ulcerative colitis
   Crohn's disease
   Radiation enterocolitis
   Ischemic colitis
   Chemotherapy-induced mucositis
   Graft-versus-host disease

Abnormal motility
   Idiopathic chronic diarrhea
   Irritable bowel syndrome
   Neoplasm (obstruction)
   Postvagotomy
   Postsurgical (e.g., gastrectomy, pyloroplasty)
   Gastroileal or gastrocolonic fistula
   Decreased rectal compliance
   Scleroderma
   Diabetic diarrhea
   Amyloidosis
Other causes/unknown/multifactorial
   Portal hypertension
   Drugs (see previous Acute Diarrhea section)
   Alcohol
   Partial bowel obstruction
   Heavy metal poisoning
   Fecal incontinence (masquerading as diarrhea)
   Uremia
   Cirrhosis
   Pernicious anemia
   Pellagra
   Immunoglobulin deficiencies
   Chronic opiate abuse
   Eosinophilic gastroenteritis
   Systemic mastocytosis
   Protein-losing enteropathy
   Long-distance running

References
1. Fine KD: Diarrhea, pp. 128–152. See Bibliography, 1.
2. Ammon HV: Diarrhea, p. 87–101. See Bibliography, 2.

5-G. Maldigestion and Malabsorption Syndromes

Maldigestion Syndromes
Pancreatic disorders
   Chronic pancreatitis
   Pancreatic resection
   Pancreatic carcinoma
   Cystic fibrosis
   Nonbeta islet cell tumors
   Severe protein malnutrition

Effect of vagotomy on pancreatic secretion
Hepatobiliary disease
    Extrahepatic biliary obstruction
    Chronic intrahepatic cholestasis (e.g., primary biliary
        cirrhosis)
    Severe hepatocellular injury
Impaired enzyme or bile salt function owing to
    Inadequate mixing (e.g., after gastric/small bowel surgery)
    Low pH in small bowel (e.g., Zollinger-Ellison
        syndrome)
    Ileal resection
    Severe diffuse ileal disease (e.g., Crohn's disease)

Malabsorption Syndromes

Mucosal disease
    Celiac sprue (gluten enteropathy)
    Collagenous sprue
    Tropical sprue
Disaccharidase diseases and carbohydrate malabsorption
    Congenital enterokinase deficiencies
    Congenital glucose-galactose malabsorption
    Congenital fructose malabsorption
    Lactase deficiency
    Sucrase-isomaltase deficiency
    Trehalase deficiency
Short bowel syndrome
    Massive resection
    Enteroenteric fistulas
    Jejunoileal bypass surgery
    Gastroileal anastomosis (inadvertent)
Neoplasms
    Intestinal lymphoma
    Extraintestinal lymphoma
    Retroperitoneal malignancy
    Carcinoid syndrome
    Adenocarcinoma
    Extraintestinal carcinoma
Cardiovascular disorders
    Congestive heart failure
    Constrictive pericarditis
    Chronic mesenteric vascular insufficiency
Endocrine disorders
    Diabetes mellitus
    Hypoparathyroidism
    Hyperthyroidism

Adrenal insufficiency
Systemic disorders
 Amyloidosis
 Protein malnutrition
 Collagen-vascular disease
  Systemic lupus erythematosus
  Scleroderma
  Rheumatoid arthritis
  Vasculitis
 Polyarteritis nodosa
 Dermatitis herpetiformis
 Psoriasis
 Kohler-Dager syndrome
 Dysgammaglobulinemia, heavy-chain
 Mastocytosis
 Food allergy
Genetic disorders
 Congenital disaccharidase deficiencies and carbohydrate
   malabsorption (see Disaccharidase Diseases
   and Carbohydrate Malabsorption section)
 Abetalipoproteinemia (fat malabsorption)
 Chloridorrhea, congenital or acquired
 Magnesium deficiency
 Vitamin D–deficient rickets
 Selective vitamin B_{12} malabsorption
 Hartnup disease
 Cystinuria (amino acid malabsorption)
Inflammation/infection
 Crohn's disease
 Behçet's disease
 Eosinophilic gastroenteritis
 Radiation enteritis
 Graft-versus-host disease
 Infectious enteritis
  Bacterial
  Bacterial overgrowth
   Surgical blind loop
   Stricture, fistula
   Crohn's disease
   Small-bowel diverticula
   Hypomotility states
    Intestinal diabetic neuropathy
    Scleroderma
    Intestinal pseudo-obstruction
  Whipple's disease

Mycobacterial (*Mycobacterium tuberculosis, M. avium*
complex)
Parasitic (*Giardia, Cryptosporidia, I. belli*)
Viral (CMV, HIV)
Drugs (partial list)
Cholestyramine
Colchicine
Broad-spectrum antibiotics (e.g., neomycin)
Cytotoxic drugs
Phenindione
Methotrexate
Mefenamic acid
Alcohol
NSAIDs
Iron salts
Laxatives
Biguanides
Paraaminosalicylic acid
Other causes
Intestinal lymphangiectasia
Pernicious anemia
Iron deficiency
Protein-losing gastroenteropathy
Idiopathic steatorrhea
Paneth cell deficiency
Congenital malrotation of the intestine
Immunodeficiency
Immunoproliferative small intestinal disease

References

1. Riley SA, Marsh MN: Maldigestion and Malabsorption,
pp. 1501–1522. See Bibliography, 1.
2. Kalser MH: Malabsorption Syndromes, p. 996. See
Bibliography, 2.

5-H. Gastrointestinal Bleeding

Upper Gastrointestinal Bleeding
Inflammation
Esophageal ulcer
Gastric ulcer*
Duodenal ulcer*
Idiopathic HIV–related esophageal ulcer

Stomal ulceration
Erosive esophagitis*
Bile acid–induced esophagitis
Erosive gastritis*
Bile acid–induced gastritis
Erosive duodenitis*
Stress ulceration
Medication-induced esophagitis
NSAID–induced gastrointestinal ulceration*
Barrett's ulcer
Graft-versus-host disease
Caustic ingestion
Eosinophilic gastroenteritis
Behçet's disease
Crohn's disease
Gastric sarcoidosis
Hypertrophic gastropathy
Infection
Esophageal moniliasis
Herpes esophagitis
CMV esophagitis
CMV gastritis
H. pylori–associated gastritis
Bacterial, fungal, and viral enteritis
M. avium complex
Neoplasms
Esophageal carcinoma
Gastric carcinoma
Small-bowel carcinoma
Ampullary carcinoma
Lymphoma
Kaposi's sarcoma
Upper gastrointestinal polyps
Leiomyoma
Sarcoma
Neurofibroma
Carcinoid tumor
Hemangioma
Plasmacytoma
Metastatic neoplasms
Heterotopic pancreatic tissue
Vascular lesions
Esophageal varices*
Gastric varices
Portal hypertensive gastropathy
Duodenal varices

Ischemic enteritis
Aortoenteric fistula
Hereditary hemorrhagic telangiectasia
Angiodysplasia
Arteriovenous malformations
Vasculitis (see vasculitides listed in Lower Gastrointestinal
        Bleeding section)
Dieulafoy lesion
Gastric antral vascular ectasia (Watermelon stomach)
Other causes
  Mallory-Weiss tear*
  Esophageal rupture (Boerhaave's syndrome)
  Duodenal diverticulum
  Meckel's diverticulum
  Other gastrointestinal diverticula
  Anticoagulant therapy
  Blood diseases and coagulopathies (e.g., hemophilia,
        thrombotic thrombocytopenic purpura)
  Uremia
  Amyloidosis
  Hemobilia
  Blue rubber bleb nevus syndrome
  Epistaxis
  Hemoptysis
  Ehlers-Danlos syndrome
  Pseudoxanthoma elasticum
  Intramural hematomas
  Whipple's disease
  Celiac disease
  Gastrointestinal foreign bodies
  Gastric prolapse into duodenum
  Volvulus
  Intussusception

Lower Gastrointestinal Bleeding
Inflammation
  Ulcerative colitis/proctitis
  Crohn's disease
  Radiation colitis*
  Solitary rectal ulcer syndrome
  Stercoral ulcer
  Anal trauma
  Typhlitis
  Medication-induced ulceration (i.e., NSAIDs, chemotherapy)
  Eosinophilic colitis
  Diversion colitis

Pouchitis
Behçet's disease
Graft-versus-host disease
Infection
   Bacterial
      Pseudomembranous colitis
      Salmonella
      Shigella
      Campylobacter
      E. coli
      Vibrio
      Gonorrhea (proctitis)
      Lymphogranuloma venereum
      Tuberculosis
      Actinomycosis
      Syphilis
   Parasitic
      Ameba
      Schistosoma
      Whipworm
   Viral
      Condyloma acuminata (anal warts)
      CMV
      HSV
   Fungal
      Histoplasmosis
Neoplasms
   Colon polyps*
   Carcinoma of the colon and rectum*
   Carcinoma of the anus
   Familial adenomatous polyposis
   Gardner's syndrome
   Peutz-Jeghers syndrome
   Juvenile polyposis
   Cronkhite-Canada syndrome
   Hamartomas
   Leiomyomas
   Leiomyosarcomas
   Kaposi's sarcoma
   Sarcomas
   Lymphomas
   Neurofibromas
   Hemangiomas
   Melanomas
   Carcinoid tumors
   Metastatic neoplasms

Vascular lesions
    Ischemic colitis*
        Mesenteric arterial thrombus
        Mesenteric arterial embolus
        Nonocclusive small bowel ischemia
    Mesenteric venous thrombosis
    Internal hemorrhoids*
    External hemorrhoids*
    Portal colopathy
    Angiodysplasia*
    Dieulafoy lesion of the colon
    Colonic varices
    Vasculitis
        Polyarteritis nodosa
        Systemic lupus erythematosus
        Rheumatoid vasculitis
        Dermatomyositis
        Stevens-Johnson syndrome
        Henoch-Schönlein purpura
        Hemolytic uremic syndrome
        Churg-Strauss syndrome
        Wegener's granulomatosis
        Essential mixed cryoglobulinemia
        Giant cell arteritis
        Köhlmeier-Degos disease
    Aortointestinal fistula
    Arteriovenous malformation
    Hereditary hemorrhagic telangiectasia
Other causes
    All upper gastrointestinal sources
    Anal fissure
    Foreign body
    Diverticulosis*
    Incarcerated hernia
    Volvulus
    Intussusception
    Prolapse of the rectum
    Uremia
    Amyloidosis
    Anticoagulation
    Blood diseases and coagulopathy
    Long-distance running
    Blue rubber bleb nevus syndrome
    Pseudoxanthoma elasticum
    Ehlers-Danlos syndrome
    Endometriosis

Colitis cystica profunda
Pneumatosis intestinalis

References

1. Laine L: Acute and Chronic Gastrointestinal Bleeding, pp. 198–219. See Bibliography, 1.
2. Katz PO, Salas L: Less Frequent Causes of Upper Gastrointestinal Bleeding. *Gastroenterol Clin North Am* 22:875–898, 1993.
3. Bogoch A: Bleeding from the Alimentary Tract, pp. 61–86. See Bibliography, 2.
4. Miller LS, Barbarevech C, Friedman LS: Less Frequent Causes of Lower Gastrointestinal Bleeding. *Gastroenterol Clin North Am* 22:21–52, 1994.

*Common causes of acute bleeding.

5-I. Abdominal Distention

Mechanical Bowel Obstruction
Extraluminal compression
    Congenital abnormalities
        Annular pancreas
        Malrotation
    Neoplasms
        Carcinomatosis
        Sarcoma
    Inflammatory disorders
        Postsurgical adhesions
        Inflammatory adhesions
        Intraabdominal abscess
    Other extraluminal causes
        Hernias
        Volvulus
        Intussusception
        Intraabdominal hematoma
        Pregnancy
        Superior mesenteric artery syndrome
Intrinsic lesions
    Congenital abnormalities
        Congenital adhesive bands
        Meckel's diverticulum
        Congenital atresia/stenosis

Duplication/cysts
Imperforate anus
Hirschsprung's disease
Neoplasms
Adenomatous polyps
Polyposis syndromes (e.g., Peutz-Jeghers syndrome)
Malignant tumors
Inflammatory disorders
Crohn's disease
Ulcerative colitis
Diverticulitis
Diverticular stricture
Tuberculosis
Endometriosis
Actinomycosis
Ischemic injury
Other intrinsic causes
Radiation stenosis
Chemical injury (potassium chloride, NSAIDs)
Bowel wall hematoma
Surgical anastomosis
Pneumatosis intestinalis
Trauma
Intraluminal contents
Foreign body
Gallstone (gallstone ileus)
Parasites (*Ascaris*)
Fecaliths
Enteroliths
Feces
Bezoar
Food impaction
Meconium

Adynamic Ileus, Nonmechanical Obstruction

Intraabdominal causes
Peritoneal inflammation (see 5-J)
Traumatic
Postoperative
Penetrating wounds
Bacterial infections
Pneumonia
Empyema
Urosepsis
Systemic infections
Chemical irritants
Blood

    Gastric contents (perforated ulcer)
    Bile
    Pancreatic enzymes (acute pancreatitis)
  Vascular insufficiency
    Intramural strangulation (distention from mechanical ileus)
    Extramural strangulation (compression of mesenteric
        vessels)
    Mesenteric artery thrombosis or embolus
  Retroperitoneal irritation
    Retroperitoneal hemorrhage
    Psoas abscess
    Pyelonephritis
    Renal colic
    Perinephric abscess
    Pancreatitis
    Pancreatic abscess
    Cancer
    Lymphoma
Extraabdominal causes
  Toxic, metabolic
    Pneumonia
    Empyema
    Uremia
    Diabetic complications
    Porphyria
    Severe systemic infection
    Heavy metal poisoning (e.g., lead)
    Severe electrolyte imbalance (e.g., hypokalemia)
  Traumatic
    Thoracic trauma
    Retroperitoneal trauma
    Intracranial trauma
    Spinal trauma
  Drugs
    Narcotics
    Anticholinergics
    Phenothiazines
    Antihistamines
    Catecholamines
  Other
    Connective tissue diseases
    Osteomyelitis of spine
    Mechanical ventilation

Vascular Obstruction
Mesenteric artery thrombosis or embolus
Mesenteric venous thrombosis

Pseudo-Obstruction Syndromes

Excessive Intraluminal Gas
Functional bowel diseases (e.g., irritable bowel syndrome)
Aerophagia
Increased intestinal gas production

Ascites (see 5-Q)

References
1. Turnage RH, Bergen PC: Intestinal Obstruction and Ileus, pp. 1799–1807. See Bibliography, 1.
2. Livingstone AS, Sosa JL: Ileus and Obstruction, pp. 1235–1248. See Bibliography, 2.

5-J. Peritonitis

Infections
    Bacterial
        Acute bacterial peritonitis
        Spontaneous bacterial peritonitis (usually in cirrhotics with ascites)
        Secondary bacterial peritonitis (associated with perforation)
        Mycobacterial (primarily *M. tuberculosis*)
    Fungal
        Candidiasis
        Histoplasmosis
        Cryptococcosis
        Coccidioidomycosis
    Parasitic
        Schistosomiasis
        Ascariasis
        Enterobiasis
        Amebiasis
        Strongyloidiasis
    HIV–associated peritonitis (from opportunistic organisms)
Spontaneous perforation of viscus
    Boerhaave's syndrome
    Peptic ulcer disease
    Appendicitis
    Cholecystitis

Pancreatitis
Diverticulitis
Necrotizing enterocolitis
Strangulated bowel
   Small-bowel adhesion
   Incarcerated hernia
   Intussusception
   Volvulus
Gastrointestinal neoplasms
Ulcerative colitis (especially with toxic megacolon)
Crohn's disease
Ischemic bowel
Ingested foreign body
Meckel's diverticulum
Ruptured visceral abscess or cyst
   Liver
   Kidney
   Spleen
   Tuboovarian
Trauma
   Blunt trauma
   Penetrating wounds
   Surgical injury, including laparoscopic surgery
   Instrumentation
      Endoscopic perforation
      Therapeutic abortion with perforation
      Paracentesis
      Bile leak after biopsy
Neoplasms
   Primary mesothelioma
   Secondary carcinomatosis
   Pseudomyxoma peritonei
Vascular causes
   Mesenteric embolus
   Mesenteric nonocclusive ischemia
   Ischemic colitis
   Portal vein thrombosis
   Mesenteric vein thrombosis
   Vasculitis
      Systemic lupus erythematosus
      Allergic vasculitis (Henoch-Schönlein purpura)
      Köhlmeier-Degos disease
      Polyarteritis nodosa
Granulomatous peritonitis
   Parasitic infestations
   Sarcoidosis

Tumors
Crohn's disease
Starch granules
Gynecologic disorders
    Chlamydia peritonitis
    Salpingitis
    Endometriosis
    Teratoma
    Leiomyomatosis
    Dermoid cyst
Chemical irritants
    Bile
    Blood
    Gastric juice
    Barium
    Enema or douche contents
Others
    Chronic peritoneal dialysis
    Eosinophilic peritonitis
    Chylous peritonitis (see 5-Q)
    Whipple's disease
    Sclerosing peritonitis
    Peritoneal lymphangiectasis
    Peritoneal encapsulation
    Peritoneal loose bodies and peritoneal cysts
    Mesothelial hyperplasia and metaplasia
    Splenosis
    Familial Mediterranean fever

References

1. Runyon BA, Hillebrand DJ: Surgical Peritonitis and Other Diseases of the Peritoneum, Mesentery, Omentum and Diaphragm, pp. 2035–2044. See Bibliography, 1.
2. Nance FC: Diseases of the Peritoneum, Retroperitoneum, Mesentery, and Omentum, pp. 3061–3105. See Bibliography, 2.

5-K. Pancreatitis

Obstruction
    Gallstone pancreatitis
    Choledocholithiasis
    Ampullary tumors

Pancreatic tumors
Metastatic carcinoma to pancreas
Periampullary diverticulum
Choledochocele
Choledochal cyst
Duodenal cyst
Pancreatic calculi
Pancreatic duct stricture*
Pancreatic pseudocyst
Pancreatic abscess
Sclerosing cholangitis
Hypertensive sphincter of Oddi
Stenosis or fibrosis of the papilla*
Congenital/inherited disorders
Pancreas divisum*
Hereditary pancreatitis*
Cystic fibrosis*
Annular pancreas
Heterotopic pancreas
Duodenal duplication
Alpha$_1$-antitrypsin deficiency*
Toxins
Alcohol*
Methanol
Organophosphate insecticides
Scorpion venom
Occupational chemicals
Drugs
Azathioprine
6-Mercaptopurine
Thiacide diuretics
Furosemide
Ethacrynic acid
Tetracycline
Sulfonamides
Nitrofurantoin
Metronidazole
Erythromycin
Pentamidine
Didanosine
Sulfasalazine
5-Acetylsalicylic acid products
L-Asparaginase
Oral contraceptives
Corticosteroids
Estrogens

    Valproic acid
    Methyldopa
    Cimetidine
    Ranitidine
    Sulindac
    Acetaminophen
    Salicylates
    Octreotide
Metabolic disorders
    Hypertriglyceridemia
    Hypercalcemia
    Hyperparathyroidism*
Trauma
    Blunt or penetrating trauma*
    Surgical trauma
    Endoscopic retrograde cholangiopancreatography
    Endoscopic sphincterotomy
    Sphincter of Oddi manometry
Vascular causes
    Postoperative pancreatitis
    Atherosclerotic emboli
    Cardiopulmonary bypass surgery
    Malignant hypertension
    Ergotamine overdose
    Systemic lupus erythematosus
    Polyarteritis nodosa
Infections
    Bacterial
        Mycoplasma
        Campylobacter jejuni
        M. tuberculosis
        Legionella
        Leptospirosis
        M. avium complex
    Viral
        Mumps
        Rubella
        Hepatitis A, B, C
        HIV
        CMV
        Coxsackievirus B
        Epstein-Barr
        Adenovirus
        Varicella
        Echo virus
    Fungal

    Candida albicans infection
    Aspergillosis
  Parasitic
    Clonorchiasis
    Ascariasis
    Cryptosporidiosis
    Toxoplasmosis
Miscellaneous
  Penetrating gastrointestinal ulcer
  Duodenal Crohn's disease
  Protein-calorie malnutrition
  Tropical pancreatitis*
  Reye's syndrome
  Hypothermia
  Idiopathic pancreatitis*
  Posttransplantation
  Food allergy
  Chronic renal insufficiency
  Severe burns
  Long-distance running
  Bulimia
  Eosinophilic pancreatitis

References

1. Steinberg W, Tenner S: Acute Pancreatitis. *N Engl J Med* 330:1198–1210, 1994.
2. Banks PA: Acute and Chronic Pancreatitis, pp. 809–862. See Bibliography, 1.
3. Lankisch PG: Chronic Pancreatitis, pp. 2930–2958. See Bibliography, 2.

*Indicates causes of pancreatitis that frequently lead to chronic pancreatitis.

5-L. Hyperamylasemia Not Associated with Pancreatitis

Intraabdominal Disorders

Common bile duct obstruction, stones
Acute cholecystitis
Biliary endoscopy (endoscopic retrograde cannulation of pancreatic duct)
Sphincter of Oddi stenosis/spasm
Perforated ulcer

Intestinal ischemia or infarction
Intestinal obstruction
Intestinal perforation
Abdominal surgery (postoperative)
Intraabdominal hemorrhage
Afferent loop syndrome
Pregnancy
Ruptured ectopic pregnancy
Salpingitis
Ovarian cysts
Dissecting aortic aneurysm
Peritonitis
Appendicitis
Tumors (e.g., lung, ovary)
Cirrhosis
Splenic rupture

Salivary Gland Disorders
Parotitis (e.g., mumps)
Alcohol ingestion
Scorpion sting
Salivary calculi
Radiation sialoadenitis
Maxillofacial surgery

Drugs
Oxyphenbutazone
Phenylbutazone
Opiates

Miscellaneous
Chronic renal insufficiency
Salivary-type hyperamylasemia
Macroamylasemia
Cerebral trauma
Burns
Traumatic shock
Diabetic ketoacidosis
Renal transplantation
Pneumonia
Acquired bisalbuminemia
Prostatic disease
Anorexia nervosa
Acute myocardial infarction
Endoscopy
HIV

Reference
1. Banks PA: Acute and Chronic Pancreatitis, pp. 809–862. See Bibliography, 1.

5-M. Hepatomegaly

Palpable Liver without Hepatic Pathology
Normal variant
Thin or flaccid abdominal wall
Depressed right diaphragm (e.g., emphysema)
Subdiaphragmatic lesion (e.g., abscess)
Riedel's lobe

True Hepatic Enlargement
Inflammatory liver disease
   Hepatitis (see 5-O)
      Infectious
         Viral
         Schistosomiasis
         Other
      Alcoholic
      Other toxins
      Drug-induced
      Autoimmune
      Steatohepatitis
      Steatosis
      Other
   Abscess
      Pyogenic
      Amebic
   Cholangitis
      Suppurative
      Sclerosing
   Pericholangitis (especially related to ulcerative colitis)
Chronic liver disease, cirrhosis (see 5-P)
   Alcoholic
   Posthepatitic
   Postnecrotic
   Cholestatic
Metabolic disorders
   Hemochromatosis
   Alpha$_1$-antitrypsin deficiency

Wilson's disease
Cystic fibrosis
Other causes
    Extrahepatic biliary obstruction
        Choledocholithiasis
        Biliary stricture
        Pancreatitis
        Carcinoma
            Bile ducts (cholangiocarcinoma)
            Head of pancreas
            Ampulla of Vater
        External compression
    Hepatic congestion
        Congestive heart failure
        Constrictive pericarditis
        Budd-Chiari syndrome (hepatic outflow obstruction)
            Thrombosis
            Tumor
            Web (inferior vena cava)
    Veno-occlusive disease
        Jamaican herbal tea
        After bone-marrow transplantation
    Infiltrative disorders, storage diseases
        Lipid accumulation
            Fatty liver
                Alcohol
                Diabetes mellitus
                Obesity
                Severe protein malnutrition
                Nonalcoholic steatohepatitis
                Jejunoileal bypass
                Parenteral hyperalimentation
                Corticosteroids, Cushing's syndrome
                Fatty liver of pregnancy
                Massive tetracycline therapy
                Toxins (e.g., carbon tetrachloride,
                    dichlorodiphenyl-trichloroethane)
                Reye's syndrome
            Lipid storage disease (especially Gaucher's disease, Niemann-Pick disease)
        Glycogen accumulation
            Glycogen storage disease
            Diabetic glycogenosis
        Granulomatous infiltration (especially sarcoidosis, miliary tuberculosis, disseminated fungal diseases, some drug reactions)
        Myelo- and lymphoproliferative disorders

Lymphoma
Myeloid metaplasia
Multiple myeloma
Leukemia
Amyloidosis
Congenital hepatic fibrosis
Hemochromatosis
Wilson's disease
Alpha$_1$-antitrypsin deficiency
Hurler's syndrome
Neoplasms
Primary
Malignant
Hepatocellular carcinoma
Cholangiocarcinoma
Angiosarcoma
Benign
Hepatic adenoma
Hemangioma
Focal nodular hyperplasia
Adenoma
Metastatic
Pancreas
Colon
Lung
Breast
Stomach
Kidney
Esophagus
Carcinoid
Cysts
Congenital
Solitary
Polycystic
Acquired (especially echinococcal)

5-N. Jaundice

Primarily Unconjugated Hyperbilirubinemia
Increased production
Hemolysis, intravascular or extravascular (see 8-B)
Ineffective erythropoiesis
Hematomas, pulmonary embolus
Decreased hepatic uptake
Gilbert's syndrome

     Drugs
        Flavaspidic acid
        Iodinated contrast agents
        Rifampin
   Decreased cystolic binding proteins (e.g., newborn or premature infants)
   Portocaval shunt
   Prolonged fasting
Decreased glucuronidation
   Crigler-Najjar syndrome, types I and II
   Gilbert's syndrome
   Physiologic jaundice of newborn
   Breast-milk jaundice
   Hepatic parenchymal disease
   Noncirrhotic portal fibrosis

Primarily Conjugated Hyperbilirubinemia
Decreased liver excretion, intrahepatic
   Familial or hereditary disorders
      Dubin-Johnson syndrome
      Rotor syndrome
      Benign recurrent intrahepatic cholestasis
      Intrahepatic cholestasis of pregnancy
   Acquired disorders
      Hepatitis (see 5-O)
      Cirrhosis (see 5-P)
      Alcoholic liver disease
      Primary sclerosing cholangitis
      Pericholangitis
      Drugs and toxins, especially
         Chlorpromazine
         Erythromycin estolate
         Isoniazid
         Halothane
   Others
      Hepatic malignancy, primary or metastatic
      Congestive heart failure
      Shock
      Sepsis
      Toxemia of pregnancy
      Hepatic trauma
      Sarcoidosis
      Amyloidosis
      Sickle cell hepatopathy
      Postoperative jaundice
      Total parenteral nutrition

Idiopathic cholestasis associated with lymphoma
Intrahepatic biliary obstruction
    Primary biliary cirrhosis
    Primary sclerosing cholangitis
    Liver allograft rejection
    Graft-versus-host disease
    Ductopenic syndromes (e.g., Alagille's
      syndrome)
    Neoplasms (primary, metastatic, lymphoma)
Extrahepatic biliary obstruction
  Congenital
    Biliary atresia
    Idiopathic dilatation of common bile duct
    Cystic fibrosis
    Choledochal cysts
  Acquired
    Cholecystitis
    Common bile duct obstruction
      Choledocholithiasis
      Tumors (benign, malignant)
        Gallbladder
        Bile ducts
        Ampulla of Vater
        Pancreas
        Lymphoma
        Metastatic tumors
      External compression
      Strictures
        Common bile duct
        Sphincter of Oddi
        Primary sclerosing cholangitis
        AIDS (*Cryptosporidium*)
      Pancreatitis
      Parasites (*Ascaris*)

5-O. Hepatitis, Abnormal "Liver Function Tests"

***Causes of Acute Liver Injury with Alanine Amino-
transferase or Asparate Aminotransferase >1,000 µ/L***
Acute viral hepatitis
Ischemic hepatopathy ("shock" liver)
Toxin, drug-induced (e.g., acetaminophen hepatotoxicity)
Autoimmune hepatitis (occasional)
Choledocholithiasis (initial, rare)

Causes of Chronic Hepatitis
Viral (type B or C)
Drug-induced
Wilson's disease
Alpha$_1$-antitrypsin deficiency
Autoimmune hepatitis
Alcoholic hepatitis

Infection
Viral
    Hepatitis A
    Hepatitis B
    Hepatitis C
    Hepatitis D (delta, only with hepatitis B)
    Hepatitis E (underdeveloped countries)
    Hepatitis G (does not lead to chronic liver disease)
    Infectious mononucleosis (Epstein-Barr virus)
    CMV
    Varicella-zoster
    Coxsackie
    Rubella
    Measles
    Herpes simplex
    Other
Bacterial (not necessarily hepatitis, *per se*)
    Pyogenic abscesses
        Numerous aerobic and anaerobic organisms
    Hepatic dysfunction in bacterial sepsis
        E. coli
        Klebsiella pneumoniae
        Pseudomonas aeruginosa
        Proteus species
        Bacteroides species
        Staphylococcus aureus
        Aerobic and anaerobic streptococci
    Hepatic dysfunction in gram-positive infections
        Pneumococcal
        Streptococcal
        Staphylococcal
        Clostridia species
    Hepatic dysfunction in gram-negative infections
        E. coli
        Paracolon bacteria
        P. aeruginosa
        Proteus
        Bacteroides

    Aerobacter
    Klebsiella
    Enterobacteriaceae
    Salmonella
    Gonococcal
    Legionnaires' bacillus
    Other
        Brucellosis
        Typhoid fever
        Tularemia
Mycobacterial
    Tuberculosis
    Leprosy
Spirochetal
    Syphilis (congenital, secondary, or late)
    Leptospirosis
    Relapsing fever (*Borrelia* species)
Mycotic
    Histoplasmosis
    Coccidioidomycosis
    Blastomycosis
    Nocardiosis
    Cryptococcosis
    Candidiasis
    Actinomycosis
Parasitic (e.g., malaria, toxoplasmosis, amebiasis, schistoso-
            miasis, others)
Rickettsial (e.g., Q fever)

Toxins
Industrial toxins (e.g., carbon tetrachloride, yellow phospho-
            rus, trichloroethylene)
Plant toxins
    Mushrooms (e.g., *Amanita phalloides*)
    Aflatoxin

Drug-Induced Liver Disease, Including Hepatitis
Drugs implicated in the etiology of chronic liver injury
    Acetaminophen
    Aspirin
    Dantrolene
    Ethanol
    Isoniazid
    Methyldopa
    Nitrofurantoin
    Oxyphenisatin

Perhexiline maleate
Propylthiouracil
Sulfonamides
Specific classes of drugs associated with acute and/or
        chronic liver dysfunction
  Anesthetics
    Chloroform
    Halothane
    Enflurane
    Methoxyflurane
    Cyclopropane
  Analgesics, antiinflammatory agents
    Acetaminophen
    Salicylates
    Propoxyphene
    Phenylbutazone
    Indomethacin
    Ibuprofen
    Naproxen
    Sulindac
  Antibacterial agents
    Erythromycin
      Estolate
      Ethylsuccinate
      Lactobionate
    Tetracyclines
    Nitrofurantoins
    Sulfonamides
    Penicillin
    Oxacillin
    Cloxacillin
    Carbenicillin
    Chloramphenicol
    Clindamycin
  Antituberculous agents
    Isoniazid
    Rifampin
    Ethionamide
    Paraaminosalicylic acid
    Pyrazinamide
  Antifungal, antiparasitic agents
    Antimony
    Arsenic
    Thiabendazole
    Hycanthone
    5-Fluorocytosine

Quinacrine
Griseofulvin
Ketoconazole
Itraconazole
Anticonvulsants
  Phenytoin
  Valproic acid
  Trimethadione
Antihypertensives, diuretics
  Chlorothiazide
  Furosemide
  Chlorthalidone
  Methyldopa
  Hydralazine
  Captopril
Antiarrhythmic agents
  Quinidine
  Aprindine
  Procainamide
  Amiodarone
Antimetabolites
  6-Mercaptopurine
  Methotrexate
  Azathioprine
  6-Thioguanine
  Chlorambucil
  5-Fluorouracil
  Nitrogen mustard
  Cyclophosphamide
Hormones
  Androgens (e.g., methyltestosterone)
  Corticosteroids
  Estrogens
Oral hypoglycemics
  Chlorpropamide
  Tolbutamide
  Tolazamide
  Acetohexamide
  Glyburide
  Troglitazone
Antithyroid drugs
  Methimazole
  Carbimazole
  Propylthiouracil
Psychoactive agents
  Phenothiazines (especially chlorpromazine)

      Imipramine
      Benzodiazepines
      Meprobamate
      Monoamine oxidase inhibitors
      Haloperidol
      Diazepam
      Chlordiazepoxide
      Desipramine
      Amitriptyline
   Others
      Doxapram
      Cimetidine
      Ranitidine
      Perhexiline maleate
      Cinchophen
      Gold salts
      Allopurinol
      Pyridium
      Papaverine
      Oxyphenisatin
      Nicotinic acid
      Disulfiram

Others
Autoimmune hepatitis
Wilson's disease
Granulomatous hepatitis of unknown etiology
Hepatitis associated with systemic disorders
   Hyperthermia
   Cardiac failure
   Shock
   Burns
   Hyperthyroidism
   Hypoxia

5-P. Cirrhosis, Chronic Liver Disease

Alcoholic
Infectious
   Viral hepatitis (especially B and C)
   Schistosomiasis
   Other infections (uncommon; e.g., congenital syphilis, bru-
         cellosis)

Biliary
- Primary biliary cirrhosis
- Primary sclerosing cholangitis
- Secondary biliary cirrhosis (chronic extrahepatic obstruction)

Autoimmune cholangiopathy
Autoimmune chronic active hepatitis
"Cryptogenic" cirrhosis
- Posthepatitic (non-B, non-C)
- Postnecrotic

Chemical
- Toxins
  - Alcohol
  - Carbon tetrachloride
  - Dimethylnitrosamine
  - Phosphorus
  - Vinyl chloride
  - Arsenic
  - Beryllium
  - Pesticides
- Drugs
  - Halothane
  - Isoniazid
  - Methotrexate
  - Methyldopa
  - Monamine oxidase inhibitors
  - Nitrofurantoin
  - Oxyphenisatin

Congestive
- Severe chronic right heart failure
  - Tricuspid insufficiency
  - Constrictive pericarditis
  - Cor pulmonale
  - Mitral stenosis
- Hepatic vein obstruction (Budd-Chiari syndrome)
- Veno-occlusive disease

Hereditary or familial disorders
- Wilson's disease
- Cystic fibrosis
- Alpha$_1$-antitrypsin deficiency
- Hemochromatosis
- Galactosemia
- Glycogen storage diseases
- Hereditary fructose intolerance
- Tyrosinosis
- Hypervitaminosis A

Thalassemia (secondary iron overload)
Sickle cell disease
Osler-Rendu-Weber syndrome
Abetalipoproteinemia
Others
Sarcoidosis
Granulomatous cirrhosis
Congenital hepatic fibrosis
Indian childhood cirrhosis
Nutritional (e.g., jejunoileal bypass surgery)
Nonalcoholic steatohepatitis

Reference
1. Tomaiolo PP, Patwardhan RV: Consequences of Chronic
Liver Disease, p. 384. See Bibliography, 13.

5-Q. Ascites

Without Peritoneal Disease
Portal hypertension
Cirrhosis (see 5-P)
Alcoholic hepatitis
Hepatic congestion
Congestive heart failure
Tricuspid insufficiency
Constrictive pericarditis
Inferior vena cava obstruction
Hepatic vein obstruction (Budd-Chiari syndrome)
Cardiomyopathy
Portal vein occlusion
Thrombosis
Tumor
Idiopathic tropical splenomegaly
Partial nodular transformation
Hypervitaminosis A
Fulminant hepatic failure
Idiopathic
Hypoalbuminemia
Cirrhosis (see 5-P)
Nephrotic syndrome
Protein-losing enteropathy
Lymphangiectasia
Severe malnutrition

Miscellaneous
    Myxedema
    Hepatocellular carcinoma (usually with cirrhosis)
    Ovarian disease
        Tumor (Meigs' syndrome)
        Struma ovarii
        Ovarian overstimulation syndrome
    Pancreatic ascites
        Rupture of pseudocyst
        Leak from pancreatic duct
    Bile ascites
        Gallbladder rupture
        Traumatic bile leak
    Chylous ascites
        Rupture (traumatic, surgical) of abdominal lymphatics
        Congenital lymphangiectasia
        Obstructed lymphatics (especially secondary to malig-
            nancy, tuberculosis, filariasis)
        Constrictive pericarditis
        Cirrhosis
        Sarcoidosis

With Peritoneal Disease
Infection
    Mycobacterial
    Bacterial
        Primary (spontaneous bacterial peritonitis in cirrhosis)
        Secondary (ruptured viscus)
    Fungal (rare, especially candidiasis, histoplasmosis,
        cryptococcosis)
    Parasitic (rare, especially schistosomiasis, ascariasis,
        enterobiasis)
    AIDS
Neoplasm
    Primary mesothelioma
    Metastatic carcinomatosis
        Ovarian
        Pancreatic
        Gastric
        Colonic
        Lymphoma
Miscellaneous
    Peritoneal vasculitides
        Systemic lupus erythematosus
        Henoch-Schönlein purpura
        Köhlmeier-Degos disease

Eosinophilic peritonitis
Familial Mediterranean fever
Pseudomyxoma peritonei
Whipple's disease
Granulomatous peritonitis
    Foreign bodies (especially starch)
    Sarcoidosis
Gynecologic lesions (especially endometriosis, ruptured
        dermoid cyst)
Peritoneal lymphangiectasis

Reference
1. Zakim D, Boyer TD (eds): Hepatology, pp. 764–788. See
   Bibliography, 3.

Bibliography

1. Feldman M, Scharschmidt BF, Sleisenger MH (eds):
   *Sleisenger and Fordtran's Gastrointestinal and Liver
   Disease*, 6/e. Philadelphia: WB Saunders, 1997.
2. Haubrich WS, Schaffner F, Berk JE (eds): *Bockus
   Gastroenterology*, 5/e. Philadelphia: WB Saunders, 1995.
3. Zakim D, Boyer TD (eds): *Hepatology. A Textbook of Liver
   Disease*, 3/e. Philadelphia: WB Saunders, 1996.
4. Bacon BR, DiBisceglie AM: *Liver Disease: Diagnosis and
   Management*. Philadelphia: WB Saunders, 1999.
5. Yamada T (ed): *Textbook of Gastroenterology*.
   Philadelphia: JB Lippincott Co, 1991.
6. Castell DO: *The Esophagus*. Boston: Little, Brown and
   Company, 1992.

6 GENITOURINARY SYSTEM

6-A. Hematuria

Pseudohematuria (Dyes and Pigments)
Beets
Food dyes
Phenytoin
Rifampin
Pyridium
Urates
Porphyrins
Myoglobin
Free hemoglobin (intravascular hemolysis)

Renal Parenchymal Causes
Primary glomerulopathy
    Postinfectious glomerulonephritis
    Thin basement membrane disease
    Immunoglobulin A (IgA) nephropathy (Berger's disease)
    Membranoproliferative glomerulonephritis
    Focal glomerulosclerosis
    Crescentic glomerulonephritis
Multisystem and hereditary diseases
    Diabetes mellitus
    Lupus erythematosus
    Goodpasture's syndrome
    Polyarteritis nodosa, other vasculitides
    Endocarditis, shunt nephritis

Hemolytic-uremic syndrome, thrombotic thrombocytopenic
    purpura
Henoch-Schönlein purpura
Malignant hypertension
Polycystic kidney disease
Hereditary nephritis (Alport's syndrome)
Fabry's disease
Nail-patella syndrome

Other
    Exercise
    Pyelonephritis, acute
    Nephrolithiasis
    Renal cyst
    Renal trauma
    Renal neoplasm
    Coagulopathy, thrombocytopenia
    Interstitial nephritis, acute
    Analgesic nephropathy
    Sickle cell trait or disease
    Medullary sponge kidney
    Lymphomatous or leukemic infiltration
    Hydronephrosis
    Oxaluria
    Vascular anomalies, intrarenal arteriovenous fistula
    Acute febrile illnesses (e.g., malaria)
    Papillary necrosis
    Renal infarction (acute renal artery occlusion, renal vein
        thrombosis)
    Renal transplant rejection

Lower Urinary Tract Causes
Congenital anomalies (e.g., ureterocele)
Neoplasms (bladder, ureter, prostate, urethral), benign or
    malignant
Cystitis, prostatitis, urethritis
Calculi
Trauma
Foreign body
Coagulopathy
Varices (renal pelvis, ureter, bladder)
Radiation cystitis
Drugs (especially cyclophosphamide, anticoagulants)
Schistosomiasis
Genitourinary tuberculosis

Non–Urinary Tract Causes
Neoplasm of adjacent organs
Diverticulitis
Pelvic inflammatory disease
Appendicitis

Reference
1. Koenig KG, Bolton WK: Clinical Evaluation and Management
   of Hematuria and Proteinuria, p. 805. See Bibliography, 8.

6-B. Polyuria

Central diabetes insipidus (see 4-T)
Renal disease
    Nephrogenic diabetes insipidus, congenital
    Chronic renal insufficiency (especially tubulointerstitial
        disease)
    Diuretic phase of acute renal failure
    Postobstructive diuresis, partial or intermittent
        obstruction
    Hypercalcemic nephropathy
    Hypokalemic nephropathy
    Sickle cell trait or disease
    Multiple myeloma
    Amyloidosis
    Sarcoidosis
    Sjögren's syndrome
    Decreased protein intake
Osmotic diuresis
    Diabetes mellitus, poorly controlled
    Mannitol or urea administration
    Iodinated contrast dye
    Hyperalimentation
    Tube feedings
Drugs
    Alcohol
    Diuretics
    Lithium
    Demeclocycline
    Methicillin
    Gentamicin

    Amphotericin B
    Phenothiazines
    Sulfonylureas
    Phenytoin
    Propoxyphene
    Methoxyflurane
    Colchicine
    Vinblastine
    Foscarnet
    Clonidine
    Norepinephrine
    Narcotic antagonists
Water load
    Psychogenic polydipsia
    Intravenous fluid therapy
    Drug-induced polydipsia (e.g., phenothiazines, anticholin-
        ergics)
    Resorption of edema fluid

Reference
1. Berl T, Schrier RW: Disorders of Water Metabolism, p. 1.
   See Bibliography, 4.

6-C. Proteinuria

Benign/Physiologic
Fever
Exercise
Orthostatic
Contrast dye

Usually Nonnephritic
Chronic pyelonephritis
Arteriolar nephrosclerosis
Malignant hypertension
Interstitial nephritis, acute or chronic
Acute tubular necrosis
Urinary tract obstruction
Nephrolithiasis
Renal neoplasm
Renal trauma
Polycystic kidney disease

Hereditary nephritis (Alport's syndrome)
Glomerular disease, especially
    IgA nephropathy (Berger's disease)
    Crescentic glomerulonephritis
    Hemolytic-uremic syndrome
    Scleroderma
Genitourinary tuberculosis

Often Nephrotic
Primary renal disease, especially
    Minimal change disease
    Membranous glomerulopathy
    Membranoproliferative glomerulonephritis
    Focal segmental glomerulosclerosis
Systemic disease, especially
    Diabetes mellitus
    Lupus erythematosus
    Polyarteritis nodosa
    Wegener's granulomatosis
    Henoch-Schönlein purpura
    Mixed cryoglobulinemia
    Amyloidosis (primary or secondary)
    Neoplasm
        Solid tumors (especially lung, colon, stomach,
            breast)
        Hodgkin's disease, other lymphomas
        Multiple myeloma
    Sarcoidosis
    Myxedema
    Graves' disease
    Sickle cell disease
Toxins, drugs
    Gold
    Mercury
    Heroin
    Nonsteroidal antiinflammatory drugs
    Penicillamine
    Captopril
    Trimethadione and other anticonvulsants
Allergens
    Pollens
    Poison ivy and oak
    Snake venom
    Bee or insect stings
    Antitoxin (e.g., tetanus toxoid)

Infection, especially
  Bacterial (e.g., streptococcal, staphylococcal)
  Hepatitis B and C
  Cytomegalovirus (CMV)
  Epstein-Barr virus (infectious mononucleosis)
  Human immunodeficiency virus (HIV)
  Syphilis
  Malaria
  Helminthic (e.g., schistosomiasis)
  Leprosy
Miscellaneous
  Congestive heart failure
  Tricuspid insufficiency
  Constrictive pericarditis
  Preeclampsia
  Renal vein thrombosis, inferior vena cava obstruction
  Massive obesity
  Hereditary diseases, especially
    Congenital nephrotic syndrome
    Fabry's disease
    Nail-patella syndrome

References
1. Glassock RJ: The Glomerulopathies, p. 685. See Bibliography, 4.
2. See Bibliography, 5.

6-D. Glomerulopathy

Primary Renal Disease
Minimal change disease
Membranous glomerulopathy
Membranoproliferative glomerulonephritis
Focal segmental glomerulosclerosis
Crescentic glomerulonephritis
Mesangial proliferative glomerulonephritis (e.g., IgA nephropathy)

Infection
Bacterial, especially
  Streptococcal
  Endocarditis
  Shunt infection

Septicemia, especially pneumococcal or
staphylococcal
Meningitis
Viral, especially
Hepatitis B and C
Mononucleosis
Rubella
Varicella
Mumps
CMV
HIV
Syphilis
Parasitic infestation (especially malaria)
Tuberculosis

Systemic Disease
Diabetes mellitus
Lupus erythematosus
Scleroderma
Rheumatoid arthritis
Mixed connective tissue disease
Polyarteritis nodosa
Wegener's granulomatosis
Hemolytic-uremic syndrome
Thrombotic thrombocytopenic purpura
Henoch-Schönlein purpura
Mixed cryoglobulinemia
Goodpasture's syndrome
Waldenström's macroglobulinemia
Amyloidosis
Fibrillary/immunotactoid glomerulopathies
Neoplasm
Solid tumors (especially lung, stomach, colon,
breast)
Hodgkin's disease, other lymphoma
Multiple myeloma, light chain nephropathy
Sarcoidosis
Preeclampsia
Postpartum renal failure
Sickle cell disease
Hepatic cirrhosis

Drugs, Toxins
Mercury
Gold
Penicillamine

Probenecid
Heroin
Amphetamines
Trimethadione

Other
Radiation
Hereditary nephritis (Alport's syndrome)
Fabry's disease
Nail-patella syndrome
Congenital nephrotic syndrome
Renal transplant rejection

References
1. Glassock RJ: The Glomerulopathies, p. 685. See
   Bibliography, 4.
2. See Bibliography, 5.

6-E. Interstitial Nephropathy

Infection
    Bacterial (pyelonephritis, acute or chronic)
    Mycoplasmal
    Toxoplasmosis
    Leptospirosis
    Brucellosis
    Mononucleosis
    Legionnaires' disease
Urinary tract obstruction, vesicoureteral reflux
Papillary necrosis
Drugs
    Analgesics (especially aspirin, phenacetin)
    Methicillin and penicillin analogues
    Sulfonamides
    Cephalosporins
    Tetracycline
    Rifampin
    Amphotericin B
    Acyclovir
    Furosemide
    Thiazides

Nonsteroidal antiinflammatory drugs
Allopurinol
Phenytoin
Azathioprine
Lithium
Cimetidine
Warfarin
Paraaminosalicylic acid
Polymyxins
Heavy metals
Lead
Cadmium
Uranium
Copper
Beryllium
Oxalate deposition
Hereditary
Small-bowel disease or resection
Ethylene glycol intoxication
Methoxyflurane anesthesia
Uric acid deposition
Gout
Tumor lysis syndrome
Hypercalcemia
Hyperparathyroidism
Neoplasm, multiple myeloma
Milk-alkali syndrome
Sarcoidosis
Hypokalemia
Radiation
Neoplastic disease
Multiple myeloma
Light chain nephropathy
Leukemic or lymphomatous infiltration
Waldenström's macroglobulinemia
Vascular causes
Arteriolar nephrosclerosis
Renal artery stenosis
Atheroembolic disease
Sickle cell trait or disease
Hereditary causes
Hereditary nephritis
Medullary sponge kidney
Medullary cystic disease
Polycystic kidney disease

    Cystinosis
    Fabry's disease
Systemic lupus erythematosus
Mixed cryoglobulinemia
Sarcoidosis
Sjögren's syndrome
Amyloidosis
Balkan nephropathy
Transplant rejection

References

1. Eknoyan G: Acute Tubulointerstitial Nephritis, p. 1249. See
   Bibliography, 5.
2. Eknoyan G: Chronic Tubulointerstitial Nephropathies, p.
   1983. See Bibliography, 5.

6-F. Renal Tubular Acidosis

Distal (Type I)
Pyelonephritis, chronic
Obstructive uropathy
Drugs, toxins
    Amphotericin B
    Analgesics
    Toluene
    Lithium
    Cyclamate
Nephrocalcinosis, especially
    Primary hyperparathyroidism
    Vitamin D intoxication
    Primary hypercalciuria
    Medullary sponge kidney
    Hyperthyroidism
Autoimmune diseases
    Hypergammaglobulinemic states, especially
        Hyperglobulinemic purpura
        Cryoglobulinemia
        Familial hypergammaglobulinemia
    Systemic lupus erythematosus
    Sjögren's syndrome
    Thyroiditis
    Chronic active hepatitis

    Primary biliary cirrhosis
    Diffuse interstitial pulmonary fibrosis
Genetically transmitted diseases
    Sickle cell disease
    Ehlers-Danlos syndrome
    Hereditary elliptocytosis
    Fabry's disease
    Wilson's disease
    Medullary cystic disease
    Hereditary fructose intolerance
Hepatic cirrhosis
Balkan nephropathy
Oxalate nephropathy
Multiple myeloma
Renal transplantation
Idiopathic (sporadic or hereditary)

Proximal (Type II)

Primary (sporadic or hereditary)
Transient (infants)
Carbonic anhydrase deficiency (e.g., genetic or acetazo-
       lamide-induced)
Fanconi's syndrome (multiple proximal tubular defects)
    Drugs and toxins
        Outdated tetracycline
        Toluene
        Gentamicin
        Streptozotocin
        Lead
        Cadmium
        Mercury
    Multiple myeloma
    Amyloidosis
    Sjögren's syndrome
    Vitamin D–deficient, –dependent, and –resistant
        states
    Cystinosis
    Tyrosinemia
    Lowe's syndrome
    Wilson's disease
    Hereditary fructose intolerance
    Pyruvate carboxylase deficiency
    Medullary cystic disease
    Paroxysmal nocturnal hemoglobinuria
    Osteopetrosis
    Renal transplantation

Type IV
Aldosterone deficiency
    Adrenal insufficiency
    Adrenal enzyme deficiency, congenital adrenal hyperpla-
        sia, especially 21-hydroxylase deficiency
    Selective aldosterone deficiency
        Hyporeninemic hypoaldosteronism
        Diabetes
        Tubulointerstitial disease
        Nonsteroidal antiinflammatory drugs
        Cyclosporine
        HIV infection
        Sickle cell disease
        Obstructive uropathy
    Heparin
    Angiotensin-converting enzyme (ACE) inhibitors
Mineralocorticoid resistance
    Pseudohypoaldosteronism
    Obstructive uropathy
    Sickle cell disease
    Drugs (spironolactone, triamterene, amiloride)

References
1. Cogan MG, Rector FC: Acid-Base Disorders, p. 737. See
   Bibliography, 1.
2. Shapiro JI, Kaehny WD: Pathogenesis and Management
   of Metabolic Acidosis and Alkalosis, p. 130. See
   Bibliography, 4.
3. Rose, p. 572. See Bibliography, 6.

6-G. Urinary Tract Obstruction

Urethral
Congenital urethral stenosis, web, atresia
Posterior urethral valves
Inflammation or stricture
Trauma

Bladder Neck
Prostatic hypertrophy, prostatitis
Carcinoma (prostate, bladder)

Bladder infection
Trauma
Functional
  Neuropathy (peripheral neuropathy, spinal cord injury or
       trauma)
  Drugs (parasympatholytics, ganglionic blockers)

Ureteral
Ureteral-pelvic junction stricture
Intraureteral
  Clots
  Stones
  Crystals (e.g., sulfa, uric acid)
  Papillae (necrosed)
  Trauma (edema, stricture)
  Tumor
  Foreign bodies
Extraureteral
  Endometriosis
  Retroperitoneal tumor or metastases, especially
    Cervical
    Endometrial
    Ovarian
    Prostatic
    Lymphoma
    Sarcoma
  Fibrosis
    Idiopathic
    Associated with inflammation, drugs (e.g., methy-
        sergide), surgery, radiation, inflammatory
        bowel disease
  Pregnancy
  Aortic or iliac aneurysm
  Aberrant vessels
  Surgical ligation
  Retroperitoneal hemorrhage
  Lymphocele

References
1. Seifter JL, Brenner BM: Urinary Tract Obstruction, p.
   1574. See Bibliography, 2.
2. Klahr S: Obstructive Nephropathy: Pathophysiology and
   Management, p. 544. See Bibliography, 4.

6-H. Nephrolithiasis

Calcium-Containing Stones
Idiopathic
Primary hypercalciuria (absorptive, renal-leak) with or without hyperuricosuria
Hypercalcemic states (see 1-L)
    Primary hyperparathyroidism
    Malignancy
    Immobilization
    Milk-alkali syndrome
    Vitamin D excess
    Sarcoidosis
    Hyperthyroidism
Renal tubular acidosis, distal
Medullary sponge kidney
Carbonic anhydrase inhibitors (e.g., acetazolamide)
Cushing's disease or syndrome
Hypoparathyroidism
Hyperoxaluria
    Primary (congenital)
    Increased metabolic production (e.g., ethylene glycol or methoxyflurane excess)
    Increased gastrointestinal absorption
        Increased dietary intake
        Small-bowel disease or resection (e.g., jejunoileal bypass, celiac sprue, Crohn's disease)

Calcium-Magnesium-Ammonium Phosphate Stones (Struvite)
Chronic infection (usually with urea-splitting organisms, for example, *Proteus*, *Klebsiella*, *Pseudomonas*), especially associated with
    Chronic Foley catheter use
    Ileal loop

Uric Acid and/or Xanthine Stones
Gout
Leukemia, lymphoma (especially after chemotherapy)
Purine pathway enzyme deficiency states
    Lesch-Nyhan syndrome
    Glycogen storage disease
    Xanthinuria
Drugs (e.g., aspirin, probenecid)

Gastrointestinal disorders associated with chronic diarrhea
(especially with ileostomy)

Cystine Stones
Cystinuria

Reference
1. Hruska KA, Seltzer JR, Grieff M: Nephrolithiasis, p. 739.
See Bibliography, 5.

6-I. Acute Renal Failure

Prerenal azotemia
Hypovolemia
  Hemorrhage
  Gastrointestinal losses
  Sweating
  Diuretic use
  Third-spacing (e.g., intestinal ileus)
  Burns
Decreased effective circulating volume
  Cirrhosis/ascites, hepatorenal syndrome
  Nephrotic syndrome
  Cardiac causes (e.g., congestive heart failure, acute
      myocardial infarction, pericardial tamponade)
Catabolic states, for example,
  Starvation with stress
  Sepsis, serious infection
  Postsurgical state
  Steroids
  Tetracycline
Breakdown of blood in gastrointestinal tract or resorption of
    hematoma

Drugs, Toxins
Heavy metals
  Mercury
  Arsenic
  Lead
  Cadmium
  Uranium
  Bismuth

    Copper
    Platinum
Carbon tetrachloride, other organic solvents
Ethylene glycol
Pesticides
Fungicides
X-ray contrast media (iodinated)
Antibiotics
    Penicillin
    Tetracycline
    Aminoglycosides
    Cephalosporins
    Amphotericin B
    Sulfonamides
    Acyclovir
    Rifampin
    Polymyxin
Other drugs
    Nonsteroidal antiinflammatory drugs
    ACE inhibitors
    Furosemide
    Phenytoin
    Phenindione
    Methoxyflurane
    Cyclosporine
    Ethylenediaminetetraacetic acid

Ischemic Disorders
Major trauma, surgery
Massive hemorrhage, severe volume depletion
Pancreatitis
Septic shock
Crush injury
Hemolysis, transfusion reaction
Rhabdomyolysis

Glomerular/Vascular Diseases
Poststreptococcal glomerulonephritis
Systemic lupus erythematosus
Scleroderma
Polyarteritis nodosa, hypersensitivity angiitis
Henoch-Schönlein purpura
Bacterial endocarditis
Serum sickness

Goodpasture's syndrome
Crescentic glomerulonephritis, idiopathic
Wegener's granulomatosis
Drug-induced vasculitis
Malignant hypertension
Hemolytic-uremic syndrome
Thrombotic thrombocytopenic purpura
Abruptio placentae
Postpartum renal failure
Transplant rejection

Interstitial/Intratubular Diseases
Interstitial nephritis (see 6-E), especially
   Infection
   Drugs
   Oxalate deposition
   Hypercalcemia
   Multiple myeloma
Pyelonephritis, papillary necrosis
Hyperuricemia
Radiation

Major Vessel Diseases
Renal artery thrombi, emboli, stenosis
Renal vein or inferior vena cava thrombosis
Dissecting aneurysm (aorta with or without renal arteries)

Postrenal Causes*
Urethral obstruction
Bladder neck obstruction
Ureteral obstruction

References
1. Anderson RJ, Schrier RW: Acute Renal Failure, p. 1069.
   See Bibliography, 5.
2. Yaqoob MM, Alkhunaizi AM, Edelstein CL, Conger JD,
   Schrier RW: Acute Renal Failure: Pathogenesis,
   Diagnosis, and Management, p. 449.
   See Bibliography, 4.

*See 6-G.

6-J. Renal Failure, Reversible Factors

Infection, upper or lower urinary tract
Obstruction
Volume depletion
Drugs, toxins
Congestive heart failure
Hypertension
Pericardial tamponade
Hypercalcemia
Hyperuricemia (>15–20 mg/dL)
Hypokalemia

Reference

1. Alfrey AC, Chan L: Chronic Renal Failure: Manifestations
   and Pathogenesis, p. 507. See Bibliography, 4.

6-K. Urinary Diagnostic Indices[a]

	Prerenal azotemia	Oliguric acute renal failure
Urine osmolality (mOsm/kg H_2O)	>500	<400
Urine Na^+ (mEq/L)	<20	>40
Urine/plasma creatinine	>40	<20
Fractional excretion of Na^+ (%)[b]	<1	>2

[a]These indices are useful only in oliguric states.
[b]Fractional excretion of Na^+ =

$$\frac{(\text{urine } Na^+ \text{ concentration}) (\text{plasma creatinine concentration})}{(\text{plasma } Na^+ \text{ concentration}) (\text{urine creatinine concentration})} \times 100\%$$

Reference

1. Yaqoob MM, Alkhunaizi AM, Edelstein CL, Conger JD,
   Schrier RW: Acute Renal Failure: Pathogenesis, Diagnosis,
   and Management, p 484. See Bibliography, 4.

6-L. Chronic Renal Failure

Glomerulopathy, primary renal*
Glomerulopathy associated with systemic disease*
Interstitial disease†
Urinary tract obstruction‡
Vascular diseases
    Nephrosclerosis
    Malignant hypertension
    Cortical necrosis
    Renal artery stenosis, thrombosis, emboli
    Renal vein thrombosis, inferior vena cava thrombosis
Genetically transmitted disease
    Polycystic kidney disease
    Hereditary nephritis
    Fabry's disease
    Oxalosis
    Cystinosis
    Medullary cystic disease
    Medullary sponge kidney
    Nail-patella syndrome
    Congenital nephrotic syndrome

References
1. See Bibliography, 5.
2. See Bibliography, 4.

*See 6-D.
†See 6-E.
‡See 6-G.

6-M. Indications for Dialysis

Biochemical Criteria
Volume overload
Serum K^+ >6 mEq/L (despite medical management)
Serum HCO_3^- <10 mEq/L, pH <7.20
Blood urea nitrogen >80–100 mg/dL
Serum creatinine >8–10 mg/dL
Creatinine clearance <10–15 mL/min

Symptomatic Criteria

Central nervous system symptoms (e.g., lethargy, confusion,
      seizures, asterixis)
Gastrointestinal symptoms (e.g., nausea, vomiting)
Pericarditis
Bleeding diathesis

Miscellaneous Indications (Conditions Not Necessarily Associated with Renal Failure)

Hypercalcemia
Hypermagnesemia
Hyperuricemia
Hypernatremia
Hypothermia
Drug overdose, toxin ingestion

Reference

1. Zawada ET: Indications for Dialysis, p. 3. See
   Bibliography, 7.

6-N. Impotence

Aging
Psychogenic causes
Testicular causes (primary or secondary)
    Congenital hypogonadism (especially Froehlich's syn-
          drome, Klinefelter's syndrome, hypogonadotropic
          eunuchoidism)
    Acquired hypogonadism
        Viral orchitis
        Trauma
        Radiation
        Hepatic insufficiency
        Chronic pulmonary disease
        Chronic renal failure
        Granulomatous disease (especially leprosy)
    Testicular carcinoma
    Pituitary tumor, especially when associated with hyper-
          prolactinemia
    Pituitary insufficiency
Neurologic disease

Anterior temporal lobe lesion
Spinal cord disease (e.g., multiple sclerosis)
Autonomic and peripheral polyneuropathies (e.g.,
　　　diabetic)
　Loss of sensory input
　　Tabes dorsalis
　　Dorsal root ganglia disease
　Lesions of nervi erigentes
　　Aortic bypass surgery
　　Prostatectomy
　　Rectosigmoid surgery
Drugs
　Antihypertensive agents
　　Thiazides
　　Beta blockers
　　Clonidine
　　Methyldopa
　　Guanadrel
　Antidepressants (e.g., tricyclics, monoamine oxidase
　　　inhibitors)
　Antipsychotic agents (e.g., phenothiazines, haloperidol,
　　　thioridazine)
　Central nervous system depressants (e.g., diazepam,
　　　chlordiazepoxide, barbiturates)
　Addictive drugs (e.g., heroin, methadone)
　Anticholinergic agents
　Antiandrogens (e.g., finasteride, leuprolide, spironolactone)
　Estrogens
Alcoholism
Vascular disease (e.g., Leriche syndrome)
Priapism, previous
Penile disease
　Trauma
　Peyronie's disease

Reference
1. McConnell JD, Wilson JD: Impotence, p. 286. See
　Bibliography, 2.

6-O. Menorrhagia and Nonmenstrual Vaginal Bleeding

Midcycle ovulatory bleeding (normal variant)
Inadequate corpus luteum (luteal phase defect)
Uterine or endometrial disease
    Endometritis
    Endometriosis
    Uterine adenomyosis
    Endometrial polyps
    Uterine leiomyomas
    Carcinoma
    Intrauterine synechiae
    Intrauterine device
Vaginal or cervical disease
    Vaginitis, cervicitis
    Cervical scarring
    Carcinoma
Abortion
Ectopic pregnancy
Ovarian destructive lesions (e.g., tumor, chronic salpingo-
          oophoritis)
Hypothalamic or pituitary lesion (e.g., tumor, sarcoidosis)
Adrenal disease (hyper- or hypofunction)
Thyroid disease (hyper- or hypofunction)

Anovulatory Bleeding
Estrogen withdrawal bleeding
Estrogen breakthrough bleeding
    Chronic, continuous estrogen therapy
    Polycystic ovarian disease
    Estrogen-secreting ovarian tumor
Progesterone breakthrough bleeding (e.g., continuous low-
          dose oral contraceptives)
Stress, psychogenic factors

Reference
1. Carr BR, Bradshaw KD: Disorders of the Ovary and
   Female Reproductive Tract, p. 2097. See Bibliography, 2.

Bibliography

1. Brenner BM, Rector FC (eds): *Brenner and Rector's The Kidney*, 5/e. Philadelphia: WB Saunders, 1996.
2. Fauci AS, Braunwald EE, Isselbacher KJ, et al. (eds): *Harrison's Principles of Internal Medicine*, 14/e. New York: McGraw-Hill, 1998.
3. Maxwell MH, Kleeman CR, Narin RG (eds): *Clinical Disorders of Fluid and Electrolyte Metabolism*, 4/e. New York: McGraw-Hill, 1987.
4. Schrier RW (ed): *Renal and Electrolyte Disorders*, 5/ed. Philadelphia: Lippincott–Raven, 1997.
5. Schrier RW, Gottschalk CW (eds): *Diseases of the Kidney*, 6/e. Boston: Little, Brown and Company, 1997.
6. Rose BD: *Clinical Physiology of Acid-Base and Electrolyte Disorders*, 4/e. New York: McGraw-Hill, 1994.
7. Daugirdas JT, Int TS (eds): *Handbook of Dialysis*, 2/e. Boston: Little, Brown and Company, 1994.
8. Neilson EG, Couser WG (eds): *Immunologic Renal Diseases*. Philadelphia: Lippincott–Raven, 1997.

7 HEMATOLOGIC SYSTEM

7-A. Anemia: Hypoproliferative (Low Reticulocyte Count)

Nutrient Deficiency
Iron deficiency
    Chronic blood loss
    Pregnancy
    Dietary deficiency
    Malabsorption
        Subtotal gastrectomy
        Malabsorption syndromes
    Hemoglobinuria or hemosiderinuria
        Intravascular hemolysis
    Hemodialysis
Vitamin B_{12} deficiency
    Dietary deficiency (rare)
    Impaired absorption
        Insufficient intrinsic factor
            Pernicious anemia
            Gastrectomy (total or partial)
            Gastric mucosal injury (e.g., lye ingestion)
            Congenital
        Malabsorption syndromes
            Sprue, tropical or nontropical
            Ileal resection
            Regional ileitis
            Infiltrative intestinal disease (e.g., lymphoma)
            Chronic pancreatitis

        Familial selective malabsorption
        Drug-induced malabsorption
      Competitive absorption
        Diphyllobothrium latum (fish tapeworm)
        Blind-loop syndromes
    Increased requirements
      Pregnancy
      Neoplasia
Folate deficiency
    Dietary deficiency (especially in alcoholics, infants)
    Impaired absorption
      Malabsorption syndromes
        Sprue, tropical or nontropical
        Whipple's disease
        Small-intestinal resection
        Infiltrative intestinal disease (e.g., lymphoma)
        Scleroderma
        Amyloidosis
      Drug-induced malabsorption (anticonvulsants)
    Increased requirements
      Pregnancy
      Infancy
      Hemolytic anemia
      Chronic exfoliative dermatitis
      Neoplasia
      Uremia
    Impaired metabolism
      Trimethoprim
      Methotrexate
      Pyrimethamine
      Alcohol
Other nutritional deficiencies
    Vitamin A
    Pyridoxine (rare)
    Vitamin C
    Starvation
    Protein deficiency (kwashiorkor)

Anemia of Chronic Disease
Chronic infection
    Subacute bacterial endocarditis
    Osteomyelitis
    Chronic pyelonephritis
    Chronic pulmonary infection
    Tuberculosis

Chronic fungal infection
Pelvic inflammatory disease
Chronic inflammatory diseases
    Rheumatoid arthritis
    Rheumatic fever
    Systemic lupus erythematosus
    Vasculitis
    Inflammatory bowel disease
    Acquired immunodeficiency syndrome (AIDS) or human
        immunodeficiency virus (HIV) infection
Malignancy
Chronic renal disease
Chronic liver disease
Endocrine dysfunction
    Hypothyroidism
    Hyperthyroidism
    Hypogonadism
    Adrenal insufficiency
    Panhypopituitarism
    Hyperparathyroidism
Pregnancy

Bone Marrow Disorders

Congenital
    Red cell aplasia (Diamond-Blackfan anemia)
    Congenital dyserythropoietic anemias
    Hereditary sideroblastic anemias
Aplastic
    Pancytopenia (see 7-L)
    Pure red cell aplasia
        Congenital (Diamond-Blackfan anemia)
        Acquired
            Associated with thymoma, chronic lymphocytic
                leukemia, and so forth
            Drug-induced
Toxic
    Megaloblastic
        Antimetabolites (e.g., 5-fluorouracil, 6-thioguanine, 6-
            mercaptopurine, azathioprine)
    Sideroblastic (e.g., alcohol, lead, isoniazid, chloramphenicol)
    Aplastic (see 7-L)
Infiltrative, with or without fibrosis
    Infection
        Tuberculosis
        Fungal disease

Gaucher's and other lipid storage diseases
Malignancy
    Hematologic (leukemia, lymphoma, myeloma)
    Marrow metastases
Neoplastic
  Leukemia, acute and chronic
  Lymphoproliferative disorders
    Lymphoma, with marrow involvement
      Hodgkin's disease
      Non-Hodgkin's lymphoma (NHL)
    Plasma cell myeloma
    Hairy-cell leukemia
  Myeloproliferative disorders
    Agnogenic myeloid metaplasia with fibrosis
    Essential thrombocythemia
    Chronic myelogenous leukemia
  Myelodysplastic syndromes
    Refractory anemia (RA)
    RA with ringed sideroblasts
    RA with excess of blasts (RAEB)
    RAEB in transformation
    Chronic myelomonocytic leukemia

Other
Marathon runner's anemia (physiologic)

References
1. Aboulafia DM, Mitsuyasu RT: Hematologic Abnormalities in AIDS. *Hematol Oncol Clin N Am* 5:195, 1991.
2. Erslev AJ: Anemia of Chronic Renal Failure; Anemia of Endocrine Disorders; Anemia of Chronic Disorders, pp. 456, 462, 518. See Bibliography, 2.
3. Fairbanks VF, Beutler E: Iron Deficiency, p. 490. See Bibliography, 2.
4. Lee GR: The Anemia of Chronic Disorders, p. 1497. See Bibliography, 1.
5. Herbert V: Hematologic Complications of Alcoholism I, II. *Semin Hematol*, vol. 17, 1980.
6. Dressendorfer RH, Wade CE, Amsterdam EA: Development of Pseudoanemia in Marathon Runners During a 20-day Road Race. *JAMA* 246:1215, 1981.
7. See Bibliography, 3.
8. Lee GR: Inherited and Drug Induced Megaloblastic Anemia, p. 973. See Bibliography, 2.

7-B. Anemia: Hyperproliferative (Increased Reticulocyte Count)

Blood Loss

Hypersplenism

Hemolytic Anemia
Hereditary
   Membrane abnormalities
      Hereditary spherocytosis
      Hereditary elliptocytosis
      Hereditary stomatocytosis
      Acanthocytosis (abetalipoproteinemia)
      Others
   Enzyme deficiencies
      Glucose-6-phosphate dehydrogenase
      Pyruvate kinase
      Others
   Hemoglobinopathies
      Qualitative
         Sickle cell anemia
         Hemoglobin C disease
         Unstable hemoglobin disease
         Others
      Unbalanced chain synthesis
         Thalassemias
Acquired
   Nonimmune
      Traumatic
         Prosthetic valves and other cardiac abnormalities
         March hemoglobinuria
         Burns
         Ionizing irradiation
      Microangiopathic hemolytic anemia
         Disseminated intravascular coagulation
         Thrombotic thrombocytopenic purpura (TTP)
         Hemolytic uremic syndrome
         Antiphospholipid antibody syndrome
         Vasculitis
         Malignant hypertension
      Infectious agents
         Malaria

   Clostridium perfringens
   Bartonella
   Babesiosis
   Others
  Chemical agents
   Naphthalene
   Arsine
   Copper
   Chlorates
   Venoms
   Distilled water (intravenous)
   Others
  Paroxysmal nocturnal hemoglobinuria
  Hypophosphatemia
  "Spur cell" anemia (liver disease)
Immune
 Warm antibody mediated
  Incompatible blood transfusion
  Hemolytic disease of newborn
  Idiopathic
  Secondary
   Infectious
    Viral [e.g., Epstein-Barr virus, cytomegalovirus
     (CMV)]
   Collagen-vascular disorders
    Systemic lupus erythematosus
    Rheumatoid arthritis
   Malignancy
    Lymphoproliferative disorders
    Solid tumors
   Other
    Sarcoidosis
    Inflammatory bowel disease
  Drugs (many)
 Cold antibody mediated
  Idiopathic
  Secondary
   Infectious
    Viral (e.g., Epstein-Barr virus)
    Mycoplasma pneumoniae
   Malignancy
 Paroxysmal cold hemoglobinuria

References

1. Lee GR: Introduction to the Hemolytic Anemias, p. 1109. See Bibliography, 1.
2. Beutler E: Glucose-6-phosphate Dehydrogenase Deficiency, p. 564. See Bibliography, 2.
3. Packman CH, Leddy JP: Acquired Hemolytic Anemia due to Warm-Reacting Autoantibodies; Cryopathic Hemolytic Syndromes; Drug Related Immunologic Injury of Erythrocytes, pp. 677, 685, 691. See Bibliography, 2.

7-C. Polycythemia

Spurious
    Decreased plasma volume (e.g., dehydration, burns)
    "Stress" erythrocytosis (Gaisböck's syndrome)
Secondary
    Appropriate (associated with tissue hypoxia)
        Decreased arterial Po_2
            Altitude
            Chronic pulmonary disease
            Alveolar hypoventilation
            Cyanotic congenital heart disease
        Normal arterial Po_2
            Carboxyhemoglobinemia (e.g., cigarette smoking)
            Hemoglobinopathies (with an increased affinity for oxygen)
            Cobalt ingestion
    Inappropriate
        Renal disorders
            Hydronephrosis
            Renal cysts
            Renal cell carcinoma
        Endocrine disorders
            Cushing's syndrome
            Primary hyperaldosteronism
            Pheochromocytoma
            Androgen therapy
        Hepatoma
        Cerebellar hemangioblastoma
        Uterine leiomyoma
        Familial erythrocytosis
Primary
    Polycythemia rubra vera

References
1. Means, Jr. RT: Polycythemia: Erythrocytosis, p. 1538. See Bibliography, 1.
2. Erslev AJ: Erythrocyte Disorders–Erythrocytosis, p. 714. See Bibliography, 2.
3. Beutler E: Polycythemia Vera, p. 324. See Bibliography, 2.

7-D. Granulocytopenia

Infections
    Viral
        Influenza
        Infectious mononucleosis
        Infectious hepatitis
        Rubella
        Chickenpox
        Smallpox
        Poliomyelitis
        Others
    Bacterial
        Overwhelming bacteremia
        Typhoid fever
        Tularemia
        Brucellosis
    Mycobacterial
        Miliary tuberculosis
    Rickettsial
    Protozoan
        Malaria
Chemical agents, drugs, physical agents
    Predictable
        Antineoplastic agents
        Benzene
        Ionizing radiation
    Idiosyncratic
        Aminopyrine
        Phenothiazines
        Antithyroid drugs
        Sulfonamides
        Anticonvulsants
        Antibiotics
        Ethanol
        Others

Systemic illness
    Systemic lupus erythematosus
    Felty's syndrome
    AIDS or HIV infection
Hypersplenism
Nutritional
    Vitamin B_{12} or folate deficiency
    Cachexia
    Alcoholism
Bone marrow dysfunction
    Acute leukemias (aleukemic)
    Lymphoproliferative disorders
    Myelofibrosis
        Primary: myeloproliferative disorders
        Secondary
            Tumor infiltration
            Infection
    Aplastic anemia
    Myelodysplastic syndromes
Immune neutropenia
    Drug-induced
    Collagen vascular disease (systemic lupus erythematosus)
    Neoplasia
    Autoimmune neutropenia
Other
    Benign neutropenia of blacks
    Chronic idiopathic neutropenia
    Cyclic neutropenia
    Benign familial neutropenia

References
1. Dale DC: Neutropenia, p. 815. See Bibliography, 2.
2. Budman DR, Steinberg AD: Hematologic Aspects of Systemic Lupus Erythematosus. *Ann Intern Med* 86:220, 1977.
3. Aboulafia DM, Mitsuyasu RT: Hematologic Abnormalities in AIDS. *Hematol Oncol Clin N Am* 5:195, 1991.

7-E. Granulocytosis

Reactive
Infection
    Bacterial (primarily)

    Mycobacterial
    Fungal
    Rickettsial
    Viral
    Spirochetal
    Parasitic
Physical stimuli
    Exercise
    Trauma
    Seizures
Inflammation, acute and chronic
    Collagen vascular disorders
    Hypersensitivity reactions
    Gout
    Vasculitis
    Nephritis
    Inflammatory bowel disease
    Hepatitis
    Pancreatitis
    Dermatitis
Neoplasm
Tissue necrosis
    Myocardial infarction
    Gangrene
    Burns
Drugs, toxins, especially
    Corticosteroids
    Epinephrine
    Lithium
    Endotoxin
    Histamine
    Lead
    Growth factors [granulocyte colony-stimulating factor (G-CSF), granulocyte-macrophage colony-stimulating factor (GM-CSF)]
Hematologic disorders
    Hemorrhage
    Postsplenectomy, functional asplenia
    Recovery from agranulocytosis
    Hemolytic anemia
    Bone marrow infiltration (e.g., solid tumor, tuberculosis)
Metabolic disorders
    Diabetic ketoacidosis
    Cushing's syndrome
    Eclampsia

Uremia
Thyroid storm
Pregnancy

Autonomous
Myeloproliferative disorders
    Chronic myelogenous leukemia
    Polycythemia rubra vera
    Agnogenic myeloid metaplasia
    Essential thrombocythemia
Acute leukemia

Congenital Causes
Down syndrome

Reference
1. Dale DC: Neutrophilia, p. 824. See Bibliography, 2.

7-F. Lymphocytosis

Infections
    Viral
        Infectious mononucleosis
        Infectious lymphocytosis
        CMV infection
        Mumps
        Measles
        Chickenpox
        Viral hepatitis
        Others
    Bacterial
        Pertussis
        Brucellosis
        Tuberculosis
    Spirochetal
        Syphilis, secondary and congenital
    Protozoan
        Toxoplasmosis
Hematologic disorders
    Lymphocytic leukemia, acute and chronic
    NHL with marrow involvement
Drug hypersensitivity

Phenytoin
p-Aminosalicylic acid
Miscellaneous
Thyrotoxicosis
Postcardiopulmonary bypass syndrome
Serum sickness
Immune thrombocytopenic purpura
Immune hemolytic anemia

Reference
1. Kipps TJ: Lymphocytosis, p. 963. See Bibliography, 2.

7-G. Lymphocytopenia

Immunodeficiency syndromes
    AIDS or HIV infection
    Congenital immunodeficiency syndromes
        Wiskott-Aldrich syndrome
        Ataxia-telangiectasia
        DiGeorge's syndrome
    Common variable immunodeficiency
Increased lymphocyte destruction
    Radiation therapy
    Antineoplastic chemotherapy
    Antilymphocyte/antithymocyte globulin
    Corticosteroid or adrenocorticotropic hormone administra-
        tion or excess
Increased lymphocyte loss
    Thoracic duct drainage
    Intestinal lymphectasia
    Intestinal lymphatic obstruction (e.g., lymphoma)
    Whipple's disease
    Severe right-sided heart failure
        Tricuspid insufficiency
        Constrictive pericarditis
Other
    Sarcoidosis
    Advanced malignancy
    Miliary tuberculosis
    Renal failure
    Aplastic anemia
    Collagen-vascular disorders
        Systemic lupus erythematosus

Idiopathic
  Idiopathic CD4⁺ T-lymphocytopenia

References
1. Kipps TJ: Lymphocytopenia, p. 963. See Bibliography, 2.
2. Spivak JL, Bender BS, Quinn TC: Hematologic Abnormalities in the Acquired Immune Deficiency Syndrome. *Am J Med* 77:224, 1984.

7-H. Monocytosis

Infections
  Tuberculosis
  Subacute bacterial endocarditis
  Syphilis
Hematologic disorders
  Myelodysplastic syndromes
  Acute nonlymphocytic leukemia (especially acute mono-
      cytic leukemia)
  Myeloproliferative disorders
  Lymphoproliferative disorders
    Hodgkin's disease
    NHL
    Myeloma
  Malignant histiocytosis
  Postsplenectomy
  Recovery from neutropenia
    Infectious
    Drug-induced
    Postchemotherapy
    Growth factor use (GM-CSF)
  Benign familial neutropenia
Collagen-vascular disorders
  Rheumatoid arthritis
  Systemic lupus erythematosus
  Temporal arteritis
  Polyarteritis nodosa
  Polymyositis
Malignancy
  Any solid tumor
Gastrointestinal disorders
  Sprue
  Ulcerative colitis

Regional enteritis
Alcoholic liver disease
Miscellaneous
Sarcoidosis

Reference
1. Lichtman MA: Monocytosis and Monocytopenia, p. 881.
   See Bibliography, 2.

7-I. Eosinophilia

Infections
    Bacterial
        Scarlet fever
        Tuberculosis
        Leprosy
        Others
    Parasitic
        Protozoans (e.g., toxoplasmosis, amebiasis, malaria)
        Metazoans (e.g., trichinosis, filariasis, schistosomiasis)
        Arthropods (e.g., scabies)
Allergic disorders
    Hay fever
    Asthma
    Bronchopulmonary aspergillosis
    Urticaria
    Angioneurotic edema
    Serum sickness
    Food allergy
Skin disorders
    Psoriasis
    Eczema
    Erythema multiforme
    Dermatitis herpetiformis
    Exfoliative dermatitis
    Pityriasis rosea
    Ichthyosis
    Pemphigus vulgaris
    Facial granuloma
Drug reactions
Hematologic disorders
    Myeloproliferative disorders
    Lymphoproliferative disorders

    Acute nonlymphocytic leukemia
    Myelodysplastic syndromes
    Postsplenectomy
    Hypereosinophilic syndrome
Malignancy
    Advanced solid tumors
Collagen-vascular disorders
    Rheumatoid arthritis
    Polyarteritis nodosa
    Vasculitis
    Dermatomyositis
    Systemic lupus erythematosus
    Eosinophilic fasciitis
Gastrointestinal disorders
    Eosinophilic gastroenteritis
    Ulcerative colitis
    Regional enteritis
Others
    Adrenal insufficiency
    Loeffler's syndrome
    Chronic eosinophilic pneumonia
    Sarcoidosis
    Radiation therapy
    Chronic renal disease
    Familial eosinophilia
    Eosinophilia-myalgia syndrome

References

1. Wardraw AJ, Kay AB: Eosinopenia and Eosinophilia, p. 844. See Bibliography, 2.
2. Chusid MJ, et al: The Hypereosinophilic Syndrome. *Medicine* 54:1, 1975.
3. Pearson DJ, Rosenow EC: Chronic Eosinophilic Pneumonia (Carrington's): A Follow-up Study. *Mayo Clin Proc* 53:73, 1978.

7-J. Thrombocytopenia

Decreased Production
Primary hematologic disorders
    Aplastic anemia
    Acute leukemia
    Lymphoproliferative disorders

    Lymphoma
    Myeloma
    Chronic lymphocytic leukemia
   Myeloproliferative disorders
    Agnogenic myeloid metaplasia with myelofibrosis
    Chronic myelogenous leukemia (accelerated phase)
   Myelodysplastic syndromes
   Selective megakaryocytic aplasia
Bone marrow infiltration
   Solid tumor
   Infection
    Tuberculosis
    Other
   Gaucher's disease
   Osteopetrosis
Drugs
   Selective megakaryocytic suppression
    Thiazides
    Alcohol
    Estrogens
    Interferon
   Nonselective myelosuppression
    Predictable (e.g., antineoplastic chemotherapy)
    Idiosyncratic (e.g., phenylbutazone)
Cyclic thrombocytopenia
Nutritional deficiency
   Folate
   Vitamin B_{12}
   Iron (rare)
Viral infections
   Influenza
   Rubella
   Infectious mononucleosis
   Thai hemorrhagic fever
   Dengue fever
   Others
Paroxysmal nocturnal hemoglobinuria
Hereditary disorders
   Wiskott-Aldrich syndrome
   May-Hegglin anomaly
Congenital causes
   Fanconi's anemia
   Amegakaryocytic thrombocytopenia with congenital mal-
     formations
   Congenital rubella or CMV infection
   Maternal thiazide ingestion

Increased Destruction
Congenital: nonimmune
    Erythroblastosis fetalis
    Maternal preeclampsia
    Congenital viral infection
    Giant cavernous hemangioma
Congenital: immune
    Maternal drug ingestion
    Isoimmune neonatal thrombocytopenia
    Maternal autoimmune thrombocytopenic purpura
Acquired: nonimmune
    Infections
        Bacterial
            Sepsis
            Typhoid fever
        Viral
            Infectious mononucleosis
            CMV
            Herpes
        Malaria
        Rickettsial
            Rocky Mountain spotted fever
    Toxic shock syndrome
    Microangiopathic hemolytic anemia
        Disseminated intravascular coagulation
        TTP
        Hemolytic-uremic syndrome
        Vasculitis
    Drugs
    Extracorporeal circulation
    Anaphylaxis
Acquired: immune
    Drug-induced
        Quinine/quinidine
        Gold salts
        Heparin
        Thiazides
        Sulfonamides
        Indomethacin
        Others
    Neoplasia-associated
        Lymphoproliferative disorders
        Solid tumors
    Collagen-vascular disorders
        Systemic lupus erythematosus
        Rheumatoid arthritis

AIDS or HIV infection
Posttransfusion purpura
Idiopathic autoimmune thrombocytopenic purpura
    Acute
    Chronic
Sarcoidosis
Hashimoto's thyroiditis
Hyperthyroidism

Sequestration/Dilution
Hypersplenism
Hypothermia
Extracorporeal circulation
Massive blood transfusion

References
1. George J: Thrombocytopenia Due to Diminished or Defective Platelet Production, p. 1281. See Bibliography, 2.
2. George J, El-Harake M: Thrombocytopenia Due to Enhanced Platelet Destruction by Non-Immunologic and Immunologic Mechanisms, p. 1290. See Bibliography, 2.
3. George J: Thrombocytopenia: Pseudothrombocytopenia Hypersplenism, and Thrombocytopenia Associated with Massive Transfusion, pp. 1355. See Bibliography, 2.
4. Aboulafia DM, Mitsuyasu RT: Hematologic Abnormalities in AIDS. *Hematol Oncol Clin N Am* 5:195, 1991.

7-K. Thrombocytosis

Primary
Myeloproliferative disorders
    Essential thrombocythemia
    Polycythemia vera
    Chronic myelogenous leukemia
    Agnogenic myeloid metaplasia with myelofibrosis

Secondary
Chronic inflammatory disorders
    Collagen-vascular disorders
        Rheumatoid arthritis
        Polyarteritis nodosa
        Wegener's granulomatosis
        Other vasculitis

    Chronic infections
        Tuberculosis
        Osteomyelitis
        Others
    Acute infections
    Inflammatory bowel disease
        Ulcerative colitis
        Regional ileitis
    Sarcoidosis
    Hepatic cirrhosis
Malignancy
Acute hemorrhage
Iron deficiency
Hemolytic anemia
Splenectomy
Recovery from thrombocytopenia (rebound)
    Myelosuppressive drug-induced
    Vitamin B_{12} or folate deficiency
    Alcohol-induced

Reference

1. Williams WJ: Thrombocytosis, p. 1361. See Bibliography, 2.

7-L. Pancytopenia

Aplastic anemias
    Congenital
        Fanconi's anemia
    Drug- or chemical-induced, or both
        Benzene
        Chloramphenicol
        Phenylbutazone
        Gold salts
        Cytotoxic chemotherapy
        Alcohol
        Others
    Radiation exposure
    Idiopathic
    Infection
        Viral, especially hepatitis
    Immunologic
Hematologic neoplasia
    Leukemia (aleukemic)
    Lymphoproliferative disorders

Lymphoma with marrow involvement
Plasma cell myeloma
Hairy-cell leukemia
Myeloproliferative disorders
Agnogenic myeloid metaplasia with myelofibrosis
Myelodysplastic syndromes
Marrow infiltration/replacement
Infection
Tuberculosis
Fungal
Gaucher's and other lipid storage diseases
Solid tumor
Osteopetrosis
Nutritional deficiencies
Vitamin B$_{12}$
Folate
Other
Collagen vascular diseases
Systemic lupus erythematosus
Paroxysmal nocturnal hemoglobinuria
Hypersplenism
Bacterial sepsis
Viral infection
AIDS or HIV infection
Sarcoidosis

References
1. Williams DM: Pancytopenia, Aplastic Anemia, and Pure Red Cell Aplasia, p. 1449. See Bibliography, 1.
2. Shaduck RK: Aplastic Anemia, p. 238. See Bibliography, 2.

7-M. Lymphadenopathy

Benign
Infection
Bacterial (any)
Mycobacterial
Bartonella (cat-scratch disease)
Fungal
Viral
Protozoal
Rickettsial
Chlamydial

Local inflammation
    Trauma
    Dermatitis
Hypersensitivity reaction
    Serum sickness
    Drug reaction
        Phenytoin
Collagen-vascular disorders
    Systemic lupus erythematosus
    Rheumatoid arthritis
    Dermatomyositis
Endocrine disorders
    Hyperthyroidism
AIDS or HIV infection
Sarcoidosis
Other
    Mucocutaneous lymph node syndrome
    Angioimmunoblastic lymphadenopathy
    Autoimmune hemolytic anemia

Malignant
Acute leukemia
Lymphoproliferative disorders
    Lymphoma
    Plasma cell myeloma
    Chronic lymphocytic leukemia
    Hairy-cell leukemia
Myeloproliferative disorders
    Chronic myelogenous leukemia
    Agnogenic myeloid metaplasia
Solid tumors

Reference
1. McCurley TL, Greer JP: Diagnostic Approach to Malignant Disorders of Hematopoietic-Lymphoid System, p. 1827. See Bibliography, 1.

7-N. Splenomegaly

Infection
    Bacterial
    Viral

Rickettsial
Fungal
Protozoal
Inflammatory
  Collagen-vascular disorders
  Hypersensitivity reactions
    Serum sickness
    Drug reactions
Hematologic neoplasms
  Acute leukemia
  Lymphoproliferative disorders
    Lymphoma
    Chronic lymphocytic leukemia
    Hairy-cell leukemia
  Myeloproliferative diseases
  Myelodysplastic syndromes
Nonhematologic neoplasm
  Primary
  Secondary
Nonmalignant hematologic disorders
  Autoimmune hemolytic anemia
  Congenital hemolytic anemias
    Hemoglobinopathies
    Hereditary spherocytosis
  Megaloblastic anemias
  Iron-deficiency anemia
  Angioimmunoblastic lymphadenopathy
Congestive splenomegaly
  Portal hypertension
  Splenic or portal vein compression or thrombosis
  Congestive heart failure
  Budd-Chiari syndrome
Infiltrative disorders
  Gaucher's and other lipid storage diseases
  Histiocytic disorders
  Amyloidosis
  Metastatic solid tumors
Other
  AIDS or HIV infection
  Sarcoidosis
  Splenic trauma/hemorrhage
  Splenic cysts
  Splenic abscess

References

1. Chapman WC, Newman M: Disorders of the Spleen, p. 1969. See Bibliography, 1.
2. Jandl JH: The Spleen and Hypersplenism, p. 407. See Bibliography, 3.

7-O. Disorders of Hemostasis

Platelet Disorders

Quantitative platelet disorders (see 7-J)
Qualitative platelet disorders
    Congenital
        Bernard-Soulier syndrome
        Glanzmann's thrombasthenia
        Storage pool deficiencies
        von Willebrand's disease
    Acquired
        Uremia
        Myeloproliferative disorders
        Myelodysplastic syndromes
        Dysproteinemias
        Drug-induced
            Aspirin
            Nonsteroidal antiinflammatory drugs
            Dextran
            Hydroxyethyl starch
            Dipyridamole
            Sulfinpyrazone
            Others
        Extracorporeal circulation

Coagulation Disorders

Congenital
    Factor deficiencies
        VIII (hemophilia A)
        IX (hemophilia B)
        XI
        V
        VII
        X

II
Combined deficiency of vitamin K–dependent factors
Fibrinogen disorders
Afibrinogenemia
Hypofibrinogenemia
Dysfibrinogenemia
von Willebrand's disease
Acquired
Vitamin K deficiency
Malabsorption syndromes
Broad-spectrum antibiotic therapy
Cholestatic jaundice
Dietary deficiency
Hemorrhagic disease of the newborn
Oral anticoagulant use/abuse
Factor X deficiency and amyloidosis
Circulating anticoagulants
Factor VIII
Associated with hemophilia A
Autoimmune disorders
Lymphoproliferative disorders/dysproteinemias
Pregnancy
Drug therapy
Penicillin
Factor IX and others
Lupus anticoagulant
With factor II deficiency
Consumptive coagulopathies
Disseminated intravascular coagulation
Liver disease
Acquired dysfibrinogenemia
Fibrinolytic states
Heparin administration
Massive blood transfusion

References

1. Coller BS: Hereditary Qualitative Platelet Disorders, pp. 1364. See Bibliography, 2.
2. Shattil SJ, Bennett JS: Acquired Qualitative Platelet Disorders, p. 1386. See Bibliography, 2.
3. Green D: Disorders of the Vitamin K-Dependent Coagulation Factors, p. 1481. See Bibliography, 2.
4. Hayer LW: Acquired Anticoagulants, p.1485 See Bibliography, 2.
5. See Bibliography, 4.

7-P. Hypercoagulable States

Congenital
Antithrombin III deficiency
Protein C deficiency
Protein S deficiency
Homocystinuria
Dysfibrinogenemias
Hyperlipidemia

Acquired
Oral contraceptive use
Lupus anticoagulant
Myeloproliferative disorders
    Essential thrombocythemia
    Polycythemia vera
Paroxysmal nocturnal hemoglobinuria
Heparin-associated thrombocytopenia
Prothrombin complex concentrate infusion
Nephrotic syndrome
Pregnancy
Disseminated intravascular coagulation (DIC)
TTP
Malignancy (with DIC) (Trousseau's syndrome)
Sickle cell anemia
Hyperviscosity syndromes
Previous venous thrombosis
Venous trauma

References
1. Bauer KA: The Hypercoagulable State, p. 1531. See Bibliography, 2.
2. Schafer AI: The Hypercoagulable States. *Ann Intern Med* 102:814, 1985.

7-Q. Disorders of Immunoglobulin Synthesis

Hypogammaglobulinemia
Congenital
    X-linked agammaglobulinemia
    Selective IgA deficiency
    Severe combined immunodeficiency

Acquired
   Common variable immunodeficiency
   Lymphoproliferative disorders
      Plasma cell myeloma
      Lymphoma
      Chronic lymphocytic leukemia
   Radiation therapy
   Antineoplastic chemotherapy
   Associated with thymoma

Hypergammaglobulinemia
Polyclonal
   Chronic inflammatory disease
      Chronic infections
      Collagen-vascular disorders
      Malignancy
      Hepatic cirrhosis
      Chronic active hepatitis
      AIDS or HIV infection
      Inflammatory bowel disease
      Sarcoidosis
      Others
   Angioimmunoblastic lymphadenopathy
Monoclonal
   Lymphoproliferative malignancies
      Plasma cell myeloma
      NHL
      Chronic lymphocytic leukemia
      Macroglobulinemia
      Heavy chain diseases
   Amyloidosis
   Monoclonal gammopathy of undetermined significance

References
1. Rosen RS: Immunodeficiency Diseases, p. 968. See
   Bibliography, 2.
2. Baird SM: Plasma Cell Neoplasms—General
   Considerations, p. 1097. See Bibliography, 2.

Bibliography

1. Lee GR, et al (eds): *Wintrobe's Clinical Hematology*, 10/e. Philadelphia: Lippincott Williams & Wilkins, 1998.
2. Williams WJ, et al (eds): *Hematology*, 5/e. New York: McGraw-Hill, 1995.
3. Jandl JH (ed): *Blood: Textbook of Hematology*. Boston: Little, Brown and Company, 1987.
4. Ratnoff OD, Forbes CD (eds): *Disorders of Hemostasis*. Philadelphia: WB Saunders, 1991.

8 INFECTIOUS DISEASE

8-A. Fever of Unknown Origin in the United States*

Infection
Bacterial
  Bacterial endocarditis
  Sinusitis
  Osteomyelitis
  Intravascular catheter infections
  Bronchiectasis
  Relapsing mastoiditis
  Upper abdominal sources
    Cholangitis
    Cholecystitis
    Empyema of the gallbladder
    Subphrenic, pancreatic, hepatic, and splenic
        abscesses
  Lower abdominal sources
    Appendicitis
    Appendiceal abscess
    Diverticulitis
    Pelvic inflammatory disease or abscess
    Perirectal abscess
    Peritonitis
    Septic pelvic thrombophlebitis
  Genitourinary sources
    Perinephric, intrarenal abscess
    Prostatic abscess
    Pyelonephritis
    Ureteral obstruction

    Renal tuberculosis
Acute rheumatic fever
Bacteremia without primary focus, especially
    Meningococcemia
    Gonococcemia
    Salmonellosis
    Listeriosis
    Brucellosis
    Ehrlichiosis
    Borreliosis
    Yersiniosis
    Tularemia
    Leptospirosis
Tuberculosis (TB), especially *Mycobacterium tuberculosis*,
    Mycobacterium avium complex, *Mycobacterium*
    kansasii
Viral, especially Epstein-Barr virus (EBV) (infectious mono-
    nucleosis), hepatitis, coxsackie B, cytomegalovirus
    (CMV), human immunodeficiency virus (HIV), par-
    vovirus B19, dengue
Chlamydial, rickettsial (especially Q fever, psittacosis)
Parasitic, protozoan, especially
    Amebiasis
    Malaria
    Trichinosis
    Toxoplasmosis
    Pneumocystis carinii
    Babesiosis
Fungal, especially
    Histoplasmosis
    Blastomycosis
    Cryptococcosis
    Coccidiomycosis
    Sporotrichosis

Malignancy
Leukemia, lymphoma, especially Hodgkin's disease
Solid tumor, especially carcinoma of
    Kidney
    Lung
    Pancreas
    Liver
    Colon
Metastatic carcinoma
Carcinomatosis
Atrial myxoma

Collagen-Vascular Disease
Systemic lupus erythematosus
Rheumatoid arthritis
Rheumatic fever
Polyarteritis nodosa, hypersensitivity vasculitis
Wegener's granulomatosis
Temporal arteritis
Adult Still's disease
Cryoglobulinemia
Churg-Strauss vasculitis
Takayasu's arteritis

Drugs
Antibiotics, especially
    Penicillins
    Cephalosporins
    Sulfonamides
    Amphotericin B
    Quinolones
    TB therapy, especially isoniazid (INH)
Allopurinol
Phenytoin
Barbiturates
Procainamide
Quinidine
Nonsteroidal antiinflammatory therapy
Antineoplastic therapy
Interferon
H_2 blockers
Methyldopa

Other
Pulmonary emboli, multiple
Thrombophlebitis
Sarcoidosis
Hepatitis (alcoholic or granulomatous)
Inflammatory bowel disease
Whipple's disease
Thyroiditis
Thyrotoxicosis
Myelofibrosis
Serum sickness
Hemolytic states
Trauma with hematoma in closed spaces (especially peri-
        splenic, perihepatic, perivesicular)

Dissecting aneurysm
Periodic fever (especially familial Mediterranean fever)
Gout
Addison's disease
Adrenal insufficiency
Weber-Christian disease
Cyclic neutropenia
Cat scratch fever
Kikuchi disease
Postpericardotomy syndrome
Factitious fever
Habitual hyperthermia

References

1. Petersdorf RG, Beeson PB: Fever of Unexplained Origin: Report on 100 Cases. *Medicine* (Baltimore) 40:1, 1961.
2. Petersdorf RG: Fever of Unknown Origin: an Old Friend Revisited (Editorial). *Arch Intern Med* 152:21, 1992.
3. See Bibliography, 1.
4. See Bibliography, 2.
5. See Bibliography, 3.
6. See Bibliography, 8.

*Defined as temperature of >38.3°C daily for 2 to 3 weeks, with cause undiagnosed despite 1 week of intensive studies in hospital.

8-B. Most Common Organisms Causing Specific Infections

Infection	Organisms
Skin and soft tissue	
Cellulitis	
Orbital	*Streptococcus pneumoniae, Haemophilus influenzae,* group A streptococci, *Moraxella catarrhalis, Staphylococcus aureus*
Nondiabetic—extremities	Group A streptococci, *S. aureus*
Diabetic—extremities	Streptococci (groups A, C, G), *S. aureus, Escherichia coli, Proteus* spp., *Klebsiella* spp., *Enterobacter* spp., *Pseudomonas aeruginosa, Enterococcus* spp., *Clostridia* spp.
Necrotizing fasciitis	Streptococci (groups A, C, G), *Clostridia* spp. + Enterobacteriaceae
Burns	*S. aureus,* streptococci, *Enterobacter* spp., *Staphylococcus epidermidis, P. aeruginosa,* fungi, herpes simplex virus (HSV)
Wounds	
Traumatic	Polymicrobial: *S. aureus,* group A and anaerobic streptococci, Enterobacteriaceae, *Clostridium perfringens, Clostridium tetani*
Water exposure	*P. aeruginosa, Aeromonas* spp.

Continued

8-B. Most Common Organisms Causing Specific Infections (continued)

Infection	Organisms
Salt water exposure	*Vibrio vulnificus, Vibrio damsela*
Postoperative Nongenitourinary, Nongynecologic, Nongastrointestinal	*S. aureus, S. epidermidis,* group A streptococci, *Enterobacteriaceae*
Genitourinary, gynecologic, gastrointestinal	*S. aureus, S. epidermidis,* group A, B, C streptococci, *Enterobacteriaceae, Enterococcus* spp., *Bacteroides* spp., *Clostridium* spp.
Decubiti Polymicrobial	Streptococci (anaerobic and groups A, C, G), *Enterococcus* spp., *S. aureus, Enterobacteriaceae, Pseudomonas* spp., *Bacteroides* spp.
Bites—dog	*Streptococcus viridans, Pasteurella multocida, S. aureus, Eikenella corrodens, Bacteroides* spp., *Fusobacterium* spp., eugonic fermenter-4, *S. epidermidis, Capnocytophagia* spp. dysgonic fermenter-2
Bites—cat	*P. multocida, S. aureus, Bartonella henselae* (cat-scratch disease), *B. henselae* and *Bartonella quintana,* both (bacillary angiomatosis, peliosis hepatitis), *B. quintana,* only (trench fever)
Bites—human	*S. viridans, S. epidermidis, S. aureus, E. corrodens, Peptostreptococcus* spp., *Bacteroides* spp., *Haemophilus parainfluenzae, Peptococcus* spp., *Fusobacterium* spp., *Corynebacterium* spp.
Bites—tick	*Borrelia burgdorferi* (Lyme disease), *Ehrlichia chaffeensis* (human monocytic ehrlichiosis), *Ehrlichia equi,* phagocytophilia (human granulocytic ehrlichiosis), *Rickettsia rickettsi*

(Rocky Mountain spotted fever), *Babesia microti* (babesiosis) *Borrelia recurrentis* (relapsing fever), *Rickettsia conorii* (spotted fever, especially boutonneuse fever)

Respiratory Infections

Sinusitis

Acute
S. pneumoniae, H. influenzae, M. catarrhalis, group A streptococci, *S. aureus,* mixed anaerobes, viruses

Chronic
Acute plus *Bacteroides* spp., *Peptostreptococcus, Fusobacterium*

Diabetic
Acute plus *P. aeruginosa, Rhizopus* spp. (*Mucoraceae*)

Neutropenic
Acute plus *Aspergillus* spp. (especially *Fumigatus*)

Pharyngitis

Acute
Streptococci (groups A, C, G), viruses (especially Coxsackie, EBV, enterocytophatogenic human orphan virus, enterovirus, HSV I–II, HIV, human herpes virus-6), *Corynebacterium diphtheriae, Mycoplasma pneumoniae, Neisseria gonorrhoeae, Candida albicans, Chlamydia pneumoniae*

Neutropenic
Acute pharyngitis, especially *C. albicans,* HSV I–II, CMV

Bronchitis

Acute
Viral, *M. pneumoniae, C. pneumoniae, H. influenzae, S. pneumoniae, M. catarrhalis, Bordetella pertussis*

Lung abscess
Bacteroides spp., *Fusobacterium* spp., *Peptostreptococcus* spp., *Prevotella* spp., microaerophilic streptococcus, streptococcus viridans

Aspiration pneumonia
Streptococcus spp., *Bacteroides* spp., *Fusobacterium* spp., *Peptostreptococcus* spp., *Moraxella catarrhalis, Eikenella corrodens*

Continued

261

8-B. Most Common Organisms Causing Specific Infections (continued)

Infection	Organisms
Nosocomial aspiration pneumonia	Aspiration pneumonia, plus *S. aureus, Enterobacteriaceae, Candida* spp.
Pneumonia	
Community acquired pneumonia (CAP) without coexistent disease, <60 yr	*S. pneumoniae, M. pneumoniae,* respiratory viruses, especially influenzae, *Parainfluenzae,* adenovirus, respiratory syncytial virus, *H. influenzae, Legionella* spp., *C. pneumoniae, Chlamydia psittaci*
Postinfluenza pneumonia	*S. pneumoniae, H. influenzae, S. aureus* (rare)
CAP with coexistent disease, >60 yr*	*S. pneumoniae, M. pneumoniae,* respiratory viruses, especially influenzae, *H. influenzae, C. pneumoniae, Legionella* spp., *K. pneumoniae, M. catarrhalis,* anaerobic bacteria if aspiration (see Aspiration Pneumonia). *M. tuberculosis,* fungi
Important exposure history for community acquired pneumonia	*Actinomyces israelii:* (especially in aspiration of poor dentition) *Coxiella burnetii.* Q fever (livestock exposure or unpasteurized milk exposure) *Brucella* spp.: cattle, swine, goat exposure *Francisella tularensis:* rabbit, tick, and deerfly exposure *Pseudomonas pseudomallei:* melioidosis (Southeast Asia travel, exposure) *Salmonella* spp.: raw, undercooked eggs, poultry, raw cookie batter *Coccidioides immitis:* inhalation of spores in Southwest United States *Histoplasma capsulatum:* inhalation of organisms from bird droppings (bats, chickens, starlings) *Blastomyces dermatitidis:* inhalation of organisms from contaminated soil

	Yersinia pestis: rat flea, infected close human contact exposure
	Legionella spp.: inhalation of organisms from contaminated water supply systems, contaminated soil
	M. pneumoniae: high incidence in closed populations (i.e., boarding schools, college dormitories, military recruit camps)
Nosocomial pneumonia (with or without mechanical ventilation)	Aerobic gram-negative bacilli (*Enterobacter aerogenes, cloacae, P. aeruginosa, cepacia, putida, K. pneumoniae, oxytoca, Acinetobacter calcoaceticus var anitratum or lwoffi, S. aureus, Legionella* spp.)
Nosocomial pneumonia (with or without mechanical ventilation)	See nosocomial pneumonia, plus fungi [*C. albicans, Aspergillus* spp. (especially fumigatus, flavus)]
Pneumonia Immunocompromised host	*S. pneumoniae, S. aureus*, aerobic gram-negative bacilli, *Legionella* spp., *Nocardia* spp. (especially with steroid use, malignancy, lymphoma, HIV), *Cryptococcus neoformans* (inhalation of organisms from pigeon droppings in soil, HIV, malignancy, diabetes mellitus, steroid use, chemotherapy), *Aspergillus* spp. (inhalation of organisms from soil or air, malignancy, especially neutropenia, steriod use, posttransplant, chemotherapy), phycomycetes: leukemia and lymphoma, *Toxoplasma gondii* [ingestion of raw or rare meat, cat feces containing cysts of *T. gondii* (e.g., litter or sandbox exposure)]
	Viruses (especially influenza, HSV, CMV, varicella-zoster virus, adenovirus, *M. tuberculosis*)
	Fungi (especially *Candida* spp., *Aspergillus* spp.)

Continued

8-B. Most Common Organisms Causing Specific Infections (continued)

Infection	Organisms
Human immuno-deficiency virus Infection	See HIV, Pulmonary Section
Meningitis	*S. pneumoniae*, *Neisseria meningitidis*, Enterovirus, EBV, HIV, HSV II, VZV, CMV, mumps, Eastern equine, Western equine, St. Louis virus, California virus, rabies virus, lymphocytic choriomeningitis, *Borrelia burgdorferi*, *Ehrlichia* spp.
Young, elderly, and immunocompro-mised	*Listeria monocytogenes*, gram-negative bacilli, *C. neoformans*, *H. influenzae* (rare since *H. influenzae* type b vaccine), leptospirosis, cerebral malaria, trichinosis, rickettsiae, mycobacteria, amebiasis, mycoplasma, treponema pallidum (syphilis)
Brain abscess	*S. pneumoniae*, streptococci, *Bacteroides* spp., *Enterobacteriaceae*, *Propionibacterium acnes*, *S. aureus*, *Nocardia* spp.
Otitis media	*S. pneumoniae*, *H. influenzae*, *M. catarrhalis*, group A streptococci, *S. aureus*, viruses, gram-negative bacilli
Mastoiditis	*S. pneumoniae*, group A streptococci, *S. aureus*, *H. influenzae*, *P. aeruginosa*, anaerobes
Conjunctivitis	Viral (adenovirus 8 and 19), *S. aureus*, *S. pneumoniae*, *H. influenzae*, *N. gonorrhoeae*, *Chlamydia trachomatis*
Keratitis	*S. aureus*, *S. epidermidis*, *S. pneumoniae*, group A streptococci, gram-negative bacilli, *P. aeruginosa* (contact lens users), *Listeria monocytogenes* (especially in diabetic patients)
Vaginitis	*Candida* spp., *Trichomonas vaginalis*, polymicrobial (especially *Gardnerella vaginalis*, *Bacteroides* spp.)

Cervicitis, nonspecific urethritis	*N. gonorrhoeae*, *C. trachomatis*, *Mycoplasma hominis*, ureaplasma, HSV, *Mycoplasma genitalium*
Pelvic inflammatory disease	*N. gonorrhoeae*, *C. trachomatis*, *Bacteroides* spp., gram-negative bacilli, streptococci
Other urogenital sexually transmitted diseases	*Treponema pallidum* (syphilis), human papillomavirus (HPV) 6, 11, 16, 18 (anogenital warts), *Haemophilus ducreyi* (chancroid), *C. trachomatis* (lymphogranuloma venereum) *Calymmatobacterium granulomatis* (granuloma inguinale), HSV type II (genital herpes)
Prostatitis	*N. gonorrhoeae*, *C. trachomatis*, gram-negative bacilli, *P. aeruginosa* (usually chronic in males >35 years of age), *Enterococcus*, *M. Tuberculosis*, mycoplasmas, ureaplasmas
Urinary tract infection	
Cystitis	*Enterobacteriaceae* (especially *E. coli*, *Enterococcus*, *Staphylococcus saprophyticus*, *C. trachomatis*)
Pyelonephritis	*Enterobacteriaceae* (especially *E. coli*, *Klebsiella* spp., *Enterococcus* spp., *P. aeruginosa*, *Proteus mirabilis*)
Perinephric abscess	*Enterobacteriaceae* (especially *E. coli*, *Klebsiella* spp., *Enterococcus* spp., *P. aeruginosa*, *Proteus mirabilis*, *S. aureus*)
Sepsis, septic shock Nonimmunocompromised host	*S. viridans*, *S. pneumoniae*, group B streptococci, *S. aureus*, *S. epidermidis*, *E. coli*, *Enterococcus*, *Klebsiella* spp., *Proteus* spp., *P. aeruginosa*, anaerobes, *H. influenzae*, *N. meningitidis*
Hospital acquired	*Enterobacteriaceae* [especially *Enterococcus* spp., *S. aureus*, *S. epidermidis*, methicillin-resistant *S. aureus* (MRSA), vancomycin-resistant enterococcus (VRE), anaerobes, *Candida* spp.]

Continued

265

8-B. Most Common Organisms Causing Specific Infections (continued)

Infection	Organisms
Immunocompromised host, neutropenia	*Enterobacteriaceae* [especially *P. aeruginosa, E. coli, Klebsiella* spp., *S. pneumoniae, S. viridans*, coagulase-negative *Staphylococcus, S. aureus, C. albicans, Aspergillus* spp., MRSA, vancomycin-resistant enterococcus (VRE), *Listeria monocytogenes*, anaerobes, *Fusobacterium* spp. (see 8-C)]
Postsplenectomy	*S. pneumoniae, H. influenzae, N. meningitidis, B. microti*
Intravenous line infections, sepsis	Coagulase-negative staphylococcus, *S. aureus, Candida* spp., *Pseudomonas* spp., *Acinetobacter* spp., *Enterobacter* spp.
In immunocompromised hosts	Coagulase-negative staphylococcus, *S. aureus, Candida* spp., *Pseudomonas* spp., *Acinetobacter* spp., *Corynebacterium jeikeium* (JK), *Aspergillus* spp., MRSA, VRE
HIV	See 13-A
Toxic shock syndrome	*S. aureus* (toxin-mediated), beta streptococci, groups A, B, C, G
Gastroenteritis	Enteric viruses (especially rotaviruses, Norwalk virus), *Shigella* spp., *Salmonella* spp., *C. jejuni, E. coli* 0157:H7, *Clostridium difficile, Entamoeba histolytica, Vibrio cholerae, Yersinia enterocolitica, Listeria monocytogenes, Vibrio parahaemolyticus, Giardia lamblia, Cyclospora* spp., *S. aureus, Bacillus cereus*
HIV-associated	See 13-E
Peritonitis	
Secondary to bowel perforation	*E. coli, Klebsiella* spp., *Enterobacter* spp., *Enterococcus* spp., *S. viridans, Bacteroides fragilis, P. aeruginosa, Clostridium* spp., *Peptostreptococcus* spp.
Spontaneous bacterial peritonitis	*S. pneumoniae, Enterobacteriaceae* (especially *E. coli*), *Enterococcus* spp., group A streptococci, anaerobes)

Intraabdominal abscess	E. coli, Klebsiella spp., Enterobacter spp., Enterococcus spp., streptococci, Bacteroides spp., S. aureus, Clostridium spp., Peptostreptococcus spp., Peptococcus spp.
Diverticulitis	Enterobacteriaceae (especially E. coli, Klebsiella spp., Proteus spp.), enterococci, Bacteroides fragilis, Peptostreptococcus spp., Clostridium spp.
Complicated appendicitis	E. coli, P. aeruginosa, Bacteroides spp., Peptostreptococcus spp., Peptococcus spp.
Acute cholecystitis	E. coli, Klebsiella spp., Enterobacter spp., Enterococcus spp., Bacteroides spp., Fusobacterium spp., Clostridium spp.
Cholangitis	E. coli, Klebsiella spp., Enterococcus spp., Bacteroides spp., Clostridium spp.
Arthritis	
Acute monoarticular	N. gonorrhoeae, S. aureus, S. pneumoniae, B. burgdorferi
Acute polyarticular	N. gonorrhoeae, S. aureus, B. burgdorferi, N. meningitidis, secondary to syphilis, parvovirus B19, rubella virus, EBV, HIV, hepatitis B
Chronic	Mycobacteria spp., fungi, Nocardia spp., Brucella spp.
Endocarditis	
Native valve	S. viridans, S. aureus, enterococci, Streptococcus bovis, S. epidermidis, HACEK (Haemophilus parainfluenzae, Haemophilus aphrophilus, Actinobacillus, Cardiobacterium, Eikenella, Kingella), fungi, C. psittaci, C. burnetii, Brucella spp., Bartonella spp.
Early prosthetic valve (<2 months postoperative)	S. epidermidis, S. aureus, streptococci, Enterobacteriaceae, diphtheroids, fungi
Late prosthetic valve (>2 months postoperative)	S. epidermidis, S. viridans, S. aureus, S. bovis, Enterobacteriaceae, enterococci, diphtheroids, fungi

Continued

267

8-B. Most Common Organisms Causing Specific Infections (continued)

Infection	Organisms
Osteomyelitis	
Acute	*S. aureus, S. epidermidis,* group A and B streptococcus, *E. coli, Salmonella* spp., *Klebsiella* spp., *Pseudomonas* spp., *S. pneumoniae, M. tuberculosis*
Chronic	*S. aureus, Klebsiella* spp., *P. aeruginosa, Klebsiella* spp., *Enterobacter* spp.

References

1. See Bibliography, 1.
2. See Bibliography, 2.
3. See Bibliography, 6.
4. See Bibliography, 8.
5. See Bibliography, 11.

*Coexisting disease: diabetes mellitus (DM), ethanol use, chronic obstructive pulmonary disease, congenital hepatic fibrosis, cigarette use, malnutrition, chronic renal failure, liver disease, post-splenectomy.

8-C. Infections in the Immunocompromised Host

Immune system abnormalities	Infections, organisms
Neutropenia	*E. Coli, P. aeruginosa, S. aureus, S. epidermis, K. pneumoniae, Enterococcus faecalis, Enterobacter cloacae, Enterobacter aerogenes, Proteus spp., Serratia marcescens, C. jeikeium, Bacillus spp., Bacteroides spp., Capnocytophaga spp., Clostridium spp., Aeromonas spp., Streptococcus spp., Legionella spp., Leuconostoc spp., Rhodococcus equi, Candida spp., Aspergillus spp., Fusarium, zygomycetes (Mucor, Rhizopus), Pseudallescheria boydii, B. henselae, HSV, CMV, Trichosporon spp., Leptotrichia buccalis, Stomatococcus mucilaginosus*
Cell-mediated deficiency (see 13-A) HIV, AIDS, lymphoma, systemic lupus erythematosus (SLE), congenital immunodeficiencies, drugs (corticosteroids, cyclo-sporine, azathioprine, cyclo-phosphamide)	*Salmonella sp., L. monocytogenes, Legionella spp., Nocardia asteroides, Bacillus sp., Candida sp., C. neoformans, T. gondii, Cryptosporidia, HSV, VZV, CMV, M. tuberculosis, Mycobacterium avium complex, Pneumocystis carinii*
Defective chemotaxis DM, Hodgkin's disease, alcohol-ism, corticosteroid use, renal failure, SLE, Job's syndrome, lazy leukocyte syndrome	Especially *Staphylococcus spp., Streptococcus spp., Candida spp.*

Continued

8-C. Infections in the Immunocompromised Host (continued)

Immune system abnormalities	Infections, organisms
Defective neutrophil killing Chronic granulomatous disease, Myeloperoxidase deficiency, Chédiak-Higashi syndrome	Especially S. aureus, E. coli, C. albicans
B-lymphocyte defects Multiple myeloma, chronic lymphatic leukemia, burns, acquired and congenital agammaglobulinemia	S. pneumoniae, H. influenzae, N. meningitidis, N. gonorrhoeae, Salmonella sp., Campylobacter sp.
Posttransplant infections Bone marrow transplant	Coagulase-negative Staphylococcus, S. viridans, S. aureus, Corynebacterium spp., E. coli, Klebsiella spp., Enterobacter spp., P. aeruginosa, S. pneumoniae, H. influenzae, Candida spp., Aspergillus spp., Trichosporon, Fusarium, Rhizopus, HSV, CMV, EBV, VZV, P. carinii, T. gondii
Renal transplant	S. aureus, E. coli, P. aeruginosa, Candida spp., C. neoformans, L. monocytogenes, CMV, M. tuberculosis, hepatitis B and C, R. equi, human parvovirus B19
Liver transplant	S. aureus, E. faecalis, Candida spp., CMV, Aspergillus spp., E. coli, Enterobacter spp., Klebsiella sp., C. neoformans, Hepatitis B and C, Polymicrobial cholangitis and peritonitis

Heart, heart–lung transplant	*S. aureus, S. epidermidis, E. coli, Klebsiella* spp., *P. aeruginosa, N. asteroides, Aspergillus* spp., CMV, HSV, *P. carinii, C. neoformans, T. gondii*
Central nervous system (CNS) infections post-transplant	Especially *N. asteroides, L. monocytogenes, T. gondii, C. neoformans, Candida* sp., zygomycetes (*Mucor*), *A. fumigatus*, VZV (See Meningitis, brain abscess, 8-B)

References

1. Hoeprich, pp. 133–140, 838–840, 936–940, 956–960. See Bibliography, 1.
2. Kelley, pp. 1570–1575, 1584–1585, 1764–1767, 1812–1819, 1968–1973. See Bibliography, 2.
3. Schlossberg, pp. 261–278. See Bibliography, 3.
4. Mandell, pp. 2666–2686, 2709–2715, 2717–2732. See Bibliography, 8.

8-D. Antimicrobial Drugs of Choice

Organism	Drugs
GRAM-POSITIVE COCCI	
S. aureus (methicillin sensitive)	Oxacillin, nafcillin, cefazolin, clindamycin, vancomycin, trimethoprim and sulfamethoxazole (TMP/SMX)
S. aureus (methicillin resistant)	Vancomycin, TMP/SMX, doxycycline, minocycline, rifampin + quinupristine plus dalfopristin (Synercid) (depends on sensitivities)
Staphylococcus epidermidis (methicillin sensitive)	Cefazolin, oxacillin, nafcillin
S. epidermidis (methicillin resistant)	Vancomycin, TMP/SMX
Staphylococcus saprophyticus	TMP/SMX, ampicillin, fluoroquinolones (FQs)
Streptococcus viridans, S. bovis [penicillin (PCN) sensitive]	Penicillin G (PCN G), cefazolin and aminoglycoside, ceftriaxone, vancomycin
S. viridans, S. bovis (intermediate PCN sensitive)	PCN G and gentamicin
Nutritionally variant streptococcus, tolerant streptococcus	Ampicillin and gentamicin, vancomycin and gentamicin, cefazolin
S. viridans, S. bovis (PCN resistant)	PCN G and gentamicin
Enterococcus spp. (PCN or ampicillin sensitive, or both)	Ampicillin and gentamicin
Enterococcus spp. (PCN resistant)	Vancomycin and gentamicin
Enterococcus spp. (VRE)	High-dose penicillin G or ampicillin, quinupristin plus dalfopristin (Synercid), doxycycline linezolid, , (not U.S. Food and Drug Administration approved) (depends on sensitivities)
Usually Enterococcus faecium	

Streptococcus pneumoniae (PCN sensitive)	PCN G, ampicillin, cefazolin, cefuroxime, cefotaxime, ceftriaxone, erythromycin, clarithromycin, azithromycin, vancomycin
S. pneumoniae (Intermediate PCN sensitive)	Ceftriaxone, cefotaxime, high-dose PCN G, ampicillin, imipenem, vancomycin
S. pneumoniae (Intermediate PCN resistant)	Vancomycin and rifampin, high-dose cefotaxime, ceftriaxone, (if not meningeal infection), imipenem, meropenem
S. pyogenes (groups A, B, C, F, G)	PCN G, ampicillin, cefazolin
GRAM-POSITIVE BACILLI	
Corynebacterium diphtheriae	Erythromycin, clindamycin, PCN G
Corynebacterium (JK strain)	Vancomycin, PCN G and gentamicin, FQ, erythromycin
Nocardia spp.	TMP/SMX, sulfonamides, amikacin and ceftriaxone
Bacillus anthracis	PCN G, FQ, erythromycin, doxycycline
Bacillus spp.	Vancomycin, clindamycin, imipenem, FQ
Lactobacillus spp.	PCN G or ampicillin and gentamicin, clindamycin, erythromycin
Leuconostoc spp.	PCN G, ampicillin, clindamycin, erythromycin, minocycline
Listeria monocytogenes	Ampicillin or PCN G and gentamicin, TMP/SMX
GRAM-NEGATIVE COCCI	
Neisseria gonorrhoeae	Ceftriaxone, cefixime, cefpodoxime, FQ, TMP/SMX
Neisseria meningitidis	PCN G, ceftriaxone, cefotaxime, chloramphenicol, TMP/SMX
Moraxella (Branhamella) catarrhalis	Ampicillin (β-lactamase–negative only), TMP/SMX, cefuroxime, ampicillin-clavulanate, ampicillin-sulbactam, ceftriaxone, cefotaxime, clarithromycin, azithromycin

Continued

273

8-D. Antimicrobial Drugs of Choice (continued)

Organism	Drugs
GRAM-NEGATIVE BACILLI	
Campylobacter jejuni	FQ, erythromycin, doxycycline, azithromycin, clarithromycin
Haemophilus influenzae	Amoxicillin-clavulanate, ampicillin-sulbactam, cefuroxime, TMP/SMX, cefotaxime, cefriaxone, azithromycin, clarithromycin, chloramphenicol
Haemophilus ducreyi	Cefriaxone, azithromycin, erythromycin, FQ, amoxicillin-clavulanate
Escherichia coli	Ampicillin, TMP/SMX, cefazolin, cefotetan, cefoxitin, ampicillin-clavulanate, ampicillin-sulbactam, FQ, cefriaxone, mezlocillin, ticarcillin-clavulanate, gentamicin, tobramycin, cefotaxime, imipenem, meropenem
Klebsiella pneumoniae	Cefazolin, cefuroxime, cefotetan, cefoxitin
Klebsiella oxytoca	TMP/SMX, FQ, cefotaxime, cefriaxone, aztreonam, amoxicillin-clavulanate, ampicillin-sulbactam, piperacillin-tazobactam, mezlocillin, imipenem
Enterobacter aerogenes *Enterobacter cloacae*	TMP/SMX, FQ, cefotaxime
Pseudomonas aeruginosa	Cefriaxone, ticarcillin-clavulanate, mezlocillin, piperacillin-tazobactam, aztreonam, imipenem, meropenem, gentamicin, tobramycin, amikacin Ceftazidime and aminoglycosides [gentamicin or tobramycin (AG)], ticarcillin-clavulanate and AG, FQ and AG or imipenem, meropenem and AG or aztreonam
Pseudomonas cepacia *(Burkholderia cepacia)*	TMP/SMX, ceftazidime, ticarcillin-clavulanate, chloramphenicol, imipenem, meropenem

Organism	Antibiotics
Stenotrophomonas maltophilia (*Xanthomonas maltophilia*)	TMP/SMX, ticarcillin-clavulanate, chloramphenicol
Acinetobacter calcoaceticus-baumanni complex	FQ, ceftazidime, ticarcillin-clavulanate, mezlocillin, piperacillin-tazobactam, imipenem, TMP/SMX
Proteus mirabilis	Ampicillin, cefazolin, cefotaxime, ceftriaxone, cefotetan, cefoxitin, aztreonam, TMP/SMX, FQ, AG
Proteus vulgaris	Cefotaxime, ceftriaxone, ceftazidime, FQ, imipenem, ticarcillin-clavulanate, ampicillin-sulbactam, aztreonam, mezlocillin, piperacillin-tazobactam, AG piperacillin
Serratia marcescens	Cefotaxime, ceftazidime, ceftriaxone, FQ, ticarcillin-clavulanate, imipenem, aztreonam, mezlocillin, meropenem, AG, piperacillin-tazobactam
Citrobacter diversus	FQ, imipenem, TMP/SMX, cefotaxime, ceftazidime, aztreonam, meropenem
Citrobacter freundii	FQ, imipenem, TMP/SMX, AG
Providencia rettgeri, Providencia stuarti	Mezlocillin, ticarcillin, cefotaxime, ceftriaxone, FQ, aztreonam, TMP/SMX, imipenem, meropenem
Morganella morganii	FQ, mezlocillin, ticarcillin, piperacillin, cefotaxime, cefotetan, cefoxitin, TMP/SMX, ceftriaxone, aztreonam, imipenem, meropenem, ceftazidime
Bartonella henselae, Bartonella quintana	Erythromycin, doxycycline, clarithromycin, azithromycin, ciprofloxacin
Salmonella typhi	FQ, ceftriaxone, chloramphenicol, TMP/SMX, ampicillin (if ampicillin sensitive)
Shigella spp.	FQ, TMP/SMX, ampicillin
Capnocytophaga canimorsus (dysgonic fermenter-2), *Capnocytophagia ochraceum* (dysgonic fermenter-1)	Clindamycin, PCN G, amoxicillin clavulanate, ceftriaxone, cefotaxime, FQ, imipenem, cefoxitin

Continued

8-D. Antimicrobial Drugs of Choice (continued)

Organism	Drugs
Pasteurella multocida	PCN, amoxicillin-clavulanate, tetracycline, ampicillin-sulbactam, ticarcillin-clavulanate, piperacillin-tazobactam, ceftriaxone, cefotaxime, ceftazidime, chloramphenicol
Eikenella corrodens	Ampicillin, PCN, tetracycline, ampicillin-clavulanate, amoxicillin-sulbactam, TMP/SMX, FQ, doxycycline
ANAEROBES	
Anaerobic streptococci, *Peptostreptococcus* spp.	PCN G, ampicillin, metronidazole, clindamycin, cefoxitin, cefotetan, mezlocillin, ticarcillin-clavulanate, imipenem
Bacteroides fragilis group	Metronidazole, clindamycin, ampicillin-sulbactam, cefoxitin, cefotetan, ticarcillin-clavulanate, mezlocillin, piperacillin-tazobactam, imipenem, chloramphenicol
Bacteroides melaninogenicus group	Metronidazole, clindamycin, PCN G, ampicillin, cefoxitin, cefotetan, ampicillin-sulbactam, mezlocillin, imipenem, chloramphenicol, meropenem
Bacteroides bivius	Metronidazole, clindamycin, cefoxitin, cefotetan, ampicillin-sulbactam, mezlocillin, ticarcillin-clavulanate, imipenem, chloramphenicol
Clostridium perfringens	PCN G, clindamycin, chloramphenicol, imipenem, doxycycline
Clostridium tetani	Metronidazole, PCN G, doxycycline, imipenem
Clostridium difficile	Oral metronidazole, oral vancomycin, bacitracin
	Nothing by mouth (NPO): intravenous metronidazole
OTHER ORGANISMS	
Legionella spp.	Erythromycin and rifampin, azithromycin +/− rifampin, FQ +/− rifampin, clarithromycin +/− rifampin, TMP/SMX +/− rifampin, doxycycline

Mycoplasma pneumoniae	Erythromycin, clarithromycin, azithromycin, doxycycline, FQ
Chlamydia pneumoniae	Doxycycline, erythromycin, FQ, azithromycin, clarithromycin
Chlamydia trachomatis	Doxycycline, azithromycin, erythromycin, FQ, chloramphenicol
Borrelia burgdorferi	Doxycycline, amoxicillin +/– probenecid, cefuroxime-axetil, clarithromycin, ceftriaxone sodium (Rocephin), PCN G, cefotaxime (Rx depends on stage)
Babesia microti	Clindamycin and quinine
Ehrlichia chaffeensis, Ehrlichia equi, Ehrlichia phagocytophilia	Doxycycline, tetracycline, chloramphenicol
Rickettsia spp.	Doxycycline, tetracycline, FQ
Leptospira	PCN, ampicillin, doxycycline
Brucella spp.	Doxycycline and rifampin, doxycycline and gentamicin or streptomycin, TMP/SMX or gentamicin, or both, ciprofloxacin
Helicobacter pylori	Bismuth and metronidazole and tetracycline and omeprazole OR metronidazole and omeprazole and clarithromycin or amoxicillin and omeprazole and clarithromycin
Actinomyces israelii	PCN G, ampicillin, clindamycin, doxycycline, ceftriaxone
VIRUSES (see 8-D and Chapter 13)	
Influenza A	Amantadine, rimantadine
Respiratory syncytial virus	Ribavirin aerosol, intravenous immunoglobulin
Herpes simplex virus	Acyclovir, valacyclovir, famciclovir
Varicella-zoster virus	Acyclovir
Cytomegalovirus (immunocompromised host)	Ganciclovir, foscarnet, cidofovir–for retinitis only

Continued

277

8-D. Antimicrobial Drugs of Choice (continued)

Organism	Drugs
HEMORRHAGIC FEVER VIRUSES	
Hantavirus pulmonary syndrome	Ribavirin (clinical trial ongoing)
Congo-Crimean hemorrhagic fever	Ribavirin
Lassa fever	Ribavirin
FUNGI (See Chapter 13 and 8-D)	
Candida albicans	
Oral	Nystatin, clotrimazole troches, fluconazole, itraconazole
Urinary tract	Fluconazole, amphotericin B
Esophageal	Fluconazole, itraconazole, amphotericin B
Vaginal	Fluconazole, miconazole, clotrimazole, miconazole, terconazole
Sepsis	Amphotericin B, fluconazole, amphotericin B lipid complex
Peritoneal (chronic ambulatory peritoneal dialysis)	Amphotericin B intraperitoneal, fluconazole
Aspergillus spp.	
Invasive (pulmonary and extra-pulmonary)	Amphotericin B, amphotericin B lipid complex, amphotericin B cholesteryl complex, liposomal amphotericin B, amphotericin B colloidal dispersion, itraconazole
Coccidiodes immitis	Fluconazole, itraconazole, amphotericin B
Cryptococcus neoformans	Amphotericin B, fluconazole
Blastomyces dermatitidis	Itraconazole, amphotericin B, fluconazole
Histoplasma capsulatum	Amphotericin B, itraconazole

Sporothrix spp.	
Lymphocutaneous	Itraconazole, saturated solution of potassium iodide, fluconazole, ketoconazole
Extracutaneous and disseminated	Amphotericin B, itraconazole
Penicillium marneffei	
Pulmonary	Itraconazole, amphotericin B, followed by itraconazole, fluconazole
Phycomycetes mucor, *Phycomycetes absidia,* *Rhizopus*	Amphotericin B
Pseudallescheria boydii	Itraconazole, miconazole
Onychomycosis	Ketoconazole, fluconazole, itraconazole, selenium sulfide lotion
Tinea versicolor	
Tinea capitis	Terbinafine, ketoconazole, itraconazole
Tinea unguium	
Tinea corporis, Tinea cruris, *Tinea pedis*	Clotrimazole, econazole, ketoconazole cream, terbinafine, ketoconazole, fluconazole
MYCOBACTERIA (See Chapter 13 and 8-D)	
Mycobacterium tuberculosis	Isoniazid, rifampin, pyrazinamide and ethambutol or streptomycin (and pyridoxine, vitamin B₆) cycloserine, ethionamide, kanamycin, ciprofloxacin, ofloxacin, levofloxacin
Mycobacterium avium intracellular complex, pulmonary and disseminated disease	Clarithromycin + ethambutol + clofazimine + either amikacin or streptomycin or clarithromycin + ethambutol + rifabutin

References
1. See Bibliography, 1.
2. See Bibliography, 2.
3. See Bibliography, 6.
4. See Bibliography, 8.
5. See Bibliography, 11.
6. See Bibliography, 14.

8-E. Antimicrobial Prophylaxis in Surgery

Surgical procedure[a]	Recommended regimen	Alternative regimen for documented allergy
Cardiac		
Pacemaker	Cefazolin, 1 g i.v. × 1	Vancomycin, 1 g i.v. × 1
Gastrointestinal		
Esophageal, gastro-duodenal	High risk[b] only: cefazolin, 1 g i.v. × 1	Clindamycin, 900 mg i.v. × 1 and gentamicin, 1.5 mg/kg × 1 (to maximum of 150 mg)
Biliary tract	High risk[c] only: cefotetan, 1 g i.v. × 1	Clindamycin, 900 mg i.v. × 1 and gentamicin, 1.5 mg/kg × 1 (to maximum of 150 mg)
Colorectal	Cefotetan, 1 g i.v. × 1	Clindamycin, 900 mg i.v. × 1 and gentamicin, 1.5 mg/kg × 1 (to maximum of 150 mg)
Appendectomy, non-perforated	Cefotetan, 1 g i.v. × 1	Clindamycin, 900 mg × 1 and gentamicin, 1.5 mg/kg × 1 (to maximum of 150 mg)
Genitourinary		
Genitourinary	High risk[d] only: ciprofloxacin 500 mg, p.o. × 1 or ciprofloxacin 400 mg, i.v. × 1	Bactrim (SMX and TMP) 10 mg/kg, × 1 (10 mg/kg TMP based on lean body weight)
Gynecologic obstetric		
Vaginal hysterectomy	Cefotetan, 1 g i.v. q 12 × 2	Clindamycin, 900 mg i.v. q 8 × 3 and gentamicin, 6 mg/kg[f] × 1
Abdominal hysterectomy	Cefotetan, 1 g i.v. × 1	Clindamycin, 900 mg i.v. ×1 and gentamicin, 1.5 mg/kg × 1 (to maximum of 150 mg)

Continued

8-E. Antimicrobial Prophylaxis in Surgery (continued)

Surgical procedure[a]	Recommended regimen	Alternative regimen for documented allergy
Cesarean section	High risk[a] only: cefotetan, 1 g i.v. × 1 (after cord clamping)	Clindamycin, 900 mg i.v. × 1, and gentamicin, 1.5 mg/kg ×1 (to maximum of 150 mg)
Head and neck Entering oral cavity or pharynx	Cefazolin, 1 g i.v. × 1	Clindamycin, 900 mg i.v. × 1
Neurosurgery Craniotomy	Cefazolin, 1 g i.v. q 8 × 3	Vancomycin, 1 g i.v. q 12 × 2
Orthopedic Total joint replacement, internal fixation of fractures	Cefazolin, 1 g i.v. q 8 × 3 or when Foley catheter is removed. Evaluate for conversion to p.o. TMP/SMX (Bactrim) DS q 12 or nitrofurantoin macrocrystals (Macrodantin), 100 mg, b.i.d. (sulfa allergy) if therapy is continued beyond initial 3 i.v. doses	Vancomycin, 1 g i.v. q 12 × 2. Evaluate for conversion to p.o. Bactrim DS q 12 or Macrodantin, 100 mg b.i.d. (sulfa allergy) if therapy is continued beyond initial 3 i.v. doses

Thoracic		
Noncardiac	Cefazolin, 1 g i.v. × 1	Vancomycin, 1 g i.v. × 1, and gentamicin, 1.5 mg/kg × 1 (to maximum of 150 mg)
Vascular		
Arterial surgery involving the abdominal aorta, prosthesis, or groin incision	Cefazolin, 1 g i.v. q 8 × 3	Vancomycin, 1 g i.v. q 12 × 2, and gentamicin, 6 mg/kg[f] × 1
Lower extremity amputation for ischemia	Cefazolin, 1 g i.v. q 8 × 3	Vancomycin, 1 g i.v. q 12 × 2, and gentamicin, 6 mg/kg[f] × 1

DS, double strength.

[a]Refer to guidelines for patients with heart valve abnormalities.

Clarification of Recommended Regimens:

[b]Esophageal or gastroduodenal procedures: High-risk includes patients with morbid obesity, esophageal obstruction, decreased gastric acidity, or decreased gastrointestinal motility.

[c]Biliary tract procedures: High-risk includes patients with acute cholecystitis, non-functioning gall bladder, obstructive jaundice, common duct stones, or patients older than age 70 years.

[d]Genitourinary procedures: High-risk patients include patients with positive urine cultures or preoperative catheter.

[e]Cesarean section: High-risk includes patients with active labor or premature rupture of membranes (not preterm).

[f]Once-daily aminoglycoside protocol at the Stamford Hospital: 6 mg/kg of gentamicin based on adjusted body weight. Decreased renal function necessitates a lower dose of the gentamicin. Please call pharmacy for additional details.

Reference

1. Gilbert DN. *Med Lett* 39:112–114, 1997.

8-F. Noninfectious Causes
of Pulmonary Infiltrates (Pseudopneumonia)

Congestive heart failure
Pulmonary emboli
Aspiration
Chemical pneumonitis
Wegener's granulomatosis
Goodpasture's syndrome
Lung carcinoma (especially alveolar cell carcinoma)
Metastatic disease
Connective tissue diseases
Vasculitis (especially systemic lupus erythematosus lung,
              rheumatoid lung)
Fat emboli
Adult respiratory distress syndrome
Eosinophilic lung disease
Allergic bronchopulmonary aspergillosis
Bronchoalveolar cell carcinoma
Hypersensitivity pneumonitis
Drug-induced pneumonitis
Pulmonary hemorrhage
Radiation pneumonitis
Acute interstitial pneumonitis
Sarcoidosis
Antineoplastic drug-induced pneumonitis (especially
              bleomycin, busulfan, methotrexate, mitomycin,
              nitrosoureas, cyclophosphamide)

8-G. Differential Diagnosis of Noninfectious Causes of Cerebrospinal Fluid Pleocytosis

Vasculitis, Mollaret's syndrome, subarachnoid hemorrhage, chemical irritation:	Intrathecal chemotherapy, spinal anesthesia, status, post myelography, status, post seizures, Behçet's syndrome, sarcoidosis, malignancy (especially leukemia), lead encephalopathy
Drugs	Nonsteroidal antiinflammatory drugs, intravenous gamma globulin, carbamazepine, penicillins, isoniazid, ciprofloxacin, metronidazole, thymidine monophosphate, sulfamethoxazole, sulfonamides, ornithine-ketoacid transaminase-3, azathioprine

Bibliography

1. Hoeprich PD, Jordan Colin M, Ronald AR: *Infectious Diseases: a Treatise of Infectious Processes*, 5/e. Philadelphia: JB Lippincott Co, 1994.
2. Kelley WN: *Textbook of Internal Medicine*, 3/e. Philadelphia: Lippincott–Raven, 1997.
3. Schlossberg D, Shulman JA: *Differential Diagnosis of Infectious Diseases*, 1/e. Philadelphia: Williams & Wilkins, 1996.
4. Carey CF, Lee HH, Woeltje KF (eds): *The Washington Manual of Medical Therapeutics*, 29/e. Philadelphia: Lippincott–Raven, 1998.
5. Powderly WG (ed): *Manual of HIV Therapeutics*. Philadelphia: Lippincott–Raven, 1997.
6. Gilbert DN, Moellering RC, Sande MA: *The Sanford Guide to Antimicrobial Therapy*, 29/e. Hyde Park, VT: Antimicrobial Therapy, 1999.
7. Reese RE, Betts RF: *A Practical Approach to Infectious Diseases*, 4/e. New York: Little, Brown, and Company, 1996.

8. Mandell GL, Bennett JE, Dolin R: *Principles and Practices of Infectious Diseases*, 4/e. New York: Churchill Livingstone, 1995.

9. Devita VT, et al: *AIDS: Etiology, Diagnosis, Treatment and Prevention*, 4/e. Philadelphia: Lippincott–Raven, 1997.

10. Wormser GP (ed): *AIDS and Other Manifestations of HIV Infection*, 3/e. Philadelphia: Lippincott–Raven, 1998.

11. Bartlett JG: *Pocket Book of Infectious Disease Therapy*. Philadelphia: Williams & Wilkins, 1997.

12. Mandell LA, Niederman MS: *Infectious Disease Clinics of North America: Lower Respiratory Tract Infections*, vol. 12. Philadelphia: Williams & Wilkins, 1998.

13. Gold JWM, Telzak EE, White DA: *The Medical Clinics of North America: Management of the HIV-Infected Patient, Part II. Infections and Malignancies Associated with HIV Infection*, Vol. 81. Philadelphia: WB Saunders, 1997.

14. Sugar AM, Lyman Caron A: *A Practical Guide to Medically Important Fungi and the Diseases They Cause*. Philadelphia: Lippincott–Raven, 1997.

15. Dolin R, Massur H, Saag MS: *AIDS Therapy*. Philadelphia: Churchill Livingstone, 1999.

16. Cotton D, Watts DH: *The Medical Management of AIDS in Women*. New York: Wiley–Liss, 1997.

17. Bartlett JG: *1999 Medical Management of HIV Infection*. Baltimore: Johns Hopkins University, Department of Infectious Diseases, 1999.

9 INTEGUMENT

9-A. Alopecia

Nonscarring
Aging (pattern baldness)
Androgenetic alopecia (e.g., secondary to ovarian or adrenal
dysfunction)
Traction or other trauma (trichotillomania, heat exposure)
Drugs
   Cytotoxic agents
   Oral contraceptives (withdrawal)
   Amphetamines
   Anticoagulants (heparin, coumadin)
   Beta blockers
   Levodopa
   Lithium
   Colchicine
   Bromocriptine
   Thallium
   Bismuth
   Borax
   Vitamin A, retinoids
   Ethionamide
   Immunoglobulin
   Interferon
   Itraconazole
   Terfenadine
   Cholesterol-lowering agents
   Cimetidine

    Captopril
    Isoniazid
    Anticonvulsants
    Propylthiouracil
Serious systemic illness, childbirth, weight loss, other
        stresses (telogen effluvium)
Cutaneous disease
    Seborrheic dermatitis
    Eczema
    Tinea capitis
    Psoriasis
    Cosmetics, other local irritants
Lupus erythematosus
Hypothyroidism, hyperthyroidism
Hypopituitarism
Syphilis, secondary
Nutritional deficiency states (kwashiorkor, marasmus, or iron,
        zinc, or biotin deficiency)
Human immunodeficiency virus (HIV) infection
Alopecia areata
Hereditary
Congenital

Scarring
Physical and chemical agents
    Burns
    Freezing
    Mechanical trauma
    Acid, alkali
    Radiation
    "Hot comb" alopecia
Infection
    Bacterial (including pyogenic infection, tertiary syphilis,
        leprosy, lupus vulgaris)
    Fungal (e.g., ringworm)
    Viral (especially varicella-zoster, variola)
    Protozoal (leishmaniasis)
Systemic disease
    Lupus erythematosus, systemic or discoid
    Scleroderma or morphea
    Sarcoidosis
    Dermatomyositis
    Amyloidosis
    Neoplasm
        Metastatic carcinoma
        Lymphoma

Cutaneous disease
    Basal cell carcinoma
    Lichen planus
    Cicatricial pemphigoid
    Necrobiosis lipoidica diabeticorum
    Folliculitis decalvans
Congenital
Idiopathic (pseudopelade of Brocq)

References

1. Helm, pp. 5–24. See Bibliography, 2.
2. Bolognia JL, Braverman IM: Skin Manifestations of
   Internal Disease, pp. 312–315. See Bibliography, 2.
3. Sauer, pp. 279–284. See Bibliography, 3.

9-B. Erythema Multiforme

Infections
    Viral [especially herpes simplex virus (HSV), Epstein-Barr,
        Coxsackie virus, echovirus, influenza]
    Bacterial (e.g., *Yersinia, Francisella tularensis*)
    Mycoplasma pneumoniae
    Chlamydial (lymphogranuloma venereum)
    Fungal (especially histoplasmosis, coccidioidomycosis)
    Parasitic (*Trichomonas*, malaria)
Vaccines [e.g., smallpox, polio, bacille Calmette-Guérin (BCG)]
Drugs, toxins
    Antibiotics (especially penicillin, sulfonamides, tetracy-
        clines, ethosuximide)
    Metals (arsenic, mercury, gold)
    Antihistamines
    Barbiturates
    Phenytoin
    Carbamazepine
    Sulfonamides
    Nonsteroidal antiinflammatory drugs (NSAIDs)
    Codeine
    Quinine
    Hydralazine
    Salicylates
    Thiazides
    Phenylbutazone
    Phenolphthalein

Neoplasms and hematologic disorders
    Lymphoma
    Leukemia
    Carcinoma
    Multiple myeloma
    Polycythemia vera
Physical factors and contact reactions
    Radiation
    Sunlight
    Cold
    Poison oak
    Fire sponge (*Tedania ignis*)
Collagen-vascular disease
    Lupus erythematosus, systemic or discoid
    Rheumatoid arthritis
    Polyarteritis nodosa
    Wegener's granulomatosis
    Dermatomyositis
    Reiter's syndrome
Sarcoidosis
Menstruation, pregnancy
Loeffler's syndrome
Beer ingestion
Idiopathic

References

1. See Bibliography, 1.
2. Helm, pp. 165–167. See Bibliography, 2.

9-C. Erythema Nodosum

Infection
    Bacterial
        Streptococci
        Yersinia
        Cat-scratch fever
        Salmonella
        Campylobacter
        M. pneumoniae
        Tularemia
    Fungal
        Histoplasmosis
        Coccidioidomycosis

      Blastomycosis
      Trichophyton
   Tuberculosis
   Leprosy
   Leptospirosis
   Chlamydial (lymphogranuloma venereum, psittacosis)
   Viral (hepatitis)
Drugs
   Penicillins
   Sulfonamides
   Salicylates
   Iodides
   Bromides
   Oral contraceptives
Sarcoidosis
Behçet's syndrome
Leukemia, lymphoma
Radiation therapy
Inflammatory bowel disease
Idiopathic
Pregnancy

References

1. Helm, pp. 81–93. See Bibliography, 2.
2. Sauer, pp. 118–119. See Bibliography, 3.

9-D. Hirsutism and Generalized Hypertrichosis

Anorexia, malnutrition
Drugs
   Minoxidil
   Corticosteroids
   Androgenic steroids
   Progestins
   Danazol
   Phenytoin
   Cyclosporine
   Hexachlorobenzene
   Diazoxide
   Penicillamine
Endocrine disorders
   Adrenogenital syndrome
   Adrenal hyperplasia, adenoma, carcinoma

  Pituitary tumor (especially Cushing's disease, acromegaly,
      prolactin-secreting tumor)
  Polycystic ovary syndrome
  Ovarian tumor
  Hyperandrogenism, insulin resistance, acanthosis nigrans
      (HAIR-AN) syndrome
  Hypothyroidism
Central nervous system disease
  Encephalitis
  Multiple sclerosis
  Head trauma
Dermatomyositis
Hereditary or congenital conditions
  Cutaneous porphyria
  Hurler's syndrome
  Morquio's disease
  Leprechaunism
  de Lange's syndrome
  Hypertrichosis lanuginosa
Hamartomas
Idiopathic

References

1. Kovacs WJ, Wilson JD: Hirsutism and Virilization, pp.
   292–294. See Bibliography, 1.
2. See Bibliography, 4.

9-E. Maculopapular Eruption, Generalized

Drugs (especially antibiotics)
Infections
  Viral
    Rubeola (paramyxovirus)
    Rubella
    Roseola (herpesvirus-6)
    Erythema infectiosum (human parvovirus)
    Infectious mononucleosis (Epstein-Barr virus)
    Cytomegalovirus
    Hepatitis B
    Other viruses (including adeno-, entero-, reo-, arbo-,
        rhabdovirus)
    HIV (retrovirus)
    Live-virus vaccine (e.g., measles)

Bacterial, especially
    Streptococcal
    Staphylococcal
    Salmonella
    Meningococcemia, chronic
Other
    Mycoplasmal
    Syphilis, secondary
    Leptospirosis
    Rat-bite fever (*spirillum minus*)
    Rickettsial (e.g., Rocky Mountain spotted fever,
        murine, typhus)
    Psittacosis
    Toxoplasmosis
    Leprosy
    Trichinosis
Systemic lupus erythematosus
Dermatomyositis
Sarcoidosis
Pityriasis rosea
Graft-versus-host disease
Kawasaki's disease

References

1. Helm, pp. 181–187. See Bibliography, 2.
2. Goldsmith, pp. 70–73, 79. See Bibliography, 3.

9-F. Petechiae and Purpura

Platelet Disorders

Thrombocytopenia (see 7-J)
    Drugs, especially
        Cytotoxic agents
        Aspirin
        Phenytoin
        NSAIDs
        Quinidine
        Quinine
        Gold
        Ethanol
        Thiazide diuretics
        Estrogens
        Heparin

Insecticides
Disseminated intravascular coagulation
  Overwhelming infection
  Bacterial (especially meningococcal, gonococcal,
      staphylococcal, gram-negative)
    Viral (especially entero-, arbo-, adenovirus; HIV
        infection)
    Rickettsial (Rocky Mountain spotted fever, louse-
        borne typhus)
    Miliary tuberculosis
    Malaria
  Anaphylaxis
  Neoplasm (especially leukemia, lymphoma, and carci-
      noma of lung, prostate, or pancreas)
  Thrombotic thrombocytopenic purpura
Immune thrombocytopenic purpura
Posttransfusion purpura
Marrow failure
Splenic sequestration of platelets
Wiskott-Aldrich syndrome
Functional platelet disorders (e.g., Glanzmann's thrombas-
      thenia, von Willebrand's disease)
Thrombocytosis

Vascular/Extravascular Causes
Vasculitis (palpable purpura)
  Henoch-Schönlein purpura
  Polyarteritis nodosa
  Churg-Strauss syndrome
  Wegener's granulomatosis
  Lupus erythematosus
  Rheumatoid arthritis
  Subacute bacterial endocarditis
  Hepatitis B
  Serum sickness
  Cryoglobulinemia
  Sjögren's syndrome
  Hyperglobulinemic purpura
  Waldenström's macroglobulinemia
  Lymphoproliferative disorders (especially Hodgkin's dis-
      ease, lymphosarcoma)
  Drugs
    Antibiotics (penicillin, sulfonamides, tetracycline)
    Thiazides
    NSAIDs

Hydralazine
Cimetidine
Phenytoin
Allopurinol
Quinidine
Propylthiouracil
Ketoconazole
Gold
Aging
Prolonged elevated venous pressure (coughing, Valsalva maneuver) or other trauma
Steroids (endogenous or exogenous)
Amyloidosis
Cholesterol or fat embolization, or both
Ehlers-Danlos syndrome
Pseudoxanthoma elasticum
Hereditary hemorrhagic telangiectasia
Scurvy
Progressive pigmentary purpura

References

1. Handin RI: Bleeding and Thrombosis, pp. 339–340. See Bibliography, 1.
2. Handin RI: Disorders of Platelets and Vessel Wall, pp. 730–733. See Bibliography, 1.
3. Helm, pp. 83–84, 94. See Bibliography, 2.

9-G. Pruritus

Pruritus with Diagnostic Skin Lesions

Infestation (especially scabies, lice, fleas)
Xerosis (dry skin; for example, secondary to low humidity or excessive bathing)
Infection, especially bacterial, fungal, varicella
Eczematous dermatitis (e.g., atopic, contact)
Urticaria (see 9-J)
Psoriasis
Dermatitis herpetiformis
Bullous pemphigoid
Lichen planus
Miliaria
Mastocytosis
Mycosis fungoides

Pruritus without Diagnostic Skin Lesions
Infestation, especially
    Hookworm
    Onchocerciasis
    Ascariasis
    Trichinosis
Drugs
    Opiates
    Aspirin
    Estrogens, progestins, androgens
    Erythromycin
    Sulfonylureas
    Phenothiazines
    Quinidine
    Vitamin B complex
    Psoralen/ultraviolet A radiation (PUVA)
Obstructive liver disease
    Bile duct obstruction, extrahepatic
    Bile duct obstruction, intrahepatic
        Biliary cirrhosis
        Drug-induced cholestasis (oral contraceptives, phe-
            nothiazines, chlorpropamide)
        Intrahepatic cholestasis of pregnancy
Neoplasm, especially
    Lymphoma, leukemia
    Abdominal malignancy
    Central nervous system malignancy
    Paraproteinemia
    Carcinoid tumor
Polycythemia vera
Iron deficiency
Diabetes mellitus
Hyperthyroidism
Chronic renal failure (with or without secondary hyper-
            parathyroidism)
Neurodermatitis

References
1. Helm, pp. 156–160. See Bibliography, 2.
2. Greco PJ, Ende J: Pruritus. *J Gen Int Med* 7:340–349, 1992.

9-H. Pustules, Generalized

Acne vulgaris
Acne rosacea
Pyogenic infection (especially disseminated gonococcal,
      Pseudomonas, meningococcal)
Viral infection (especially vaccinia, variola)
Eosinophilic folliculitis in HIV infection
Disseminated cryptococcosis
Syphilis, secondary
Drugs, especially
    Antibiotics
    Phenytoin
    Halogens (iodide, bromide)
    Corticosteroids
    Lithium
    Isoniazid
    Diltiazem
    Furosemide
    Carbamazepine
    Androgenic steroids
    Oral contraceptives
Pustular psoriasis
Sweet's syndrome (acute febrile neutrophilic dermatosis)
Behçet's syndrome
Polycystic ovary disease
Cushing's disease, 21-hydroxylase deficiency

References
1. Helm, pp. 189–198. See Bibliography, 2.
2. Bolognia JL, Braverman IM: Skin Manifestations of
   Internal Disease, p. 315. See Bibliography, 1.
3. Webster GF: Pustular Drug Reactions. *Clin Dermatol*
   11:541–543, 1993.

9-I. Telangiectasia

Normal variant (especially with wind or sun exposure)
Endocrine disease
    Chronic liver disease (especially alcoholic cirrhosis)
    Pregnancy, estrogen, or progesterone therapy
    Topical steroid therapy (long-term)

Hyperthyroidism
Collagen-vascular disease
    Lupus erythematosus, systemic or discoid
    Dermatomyositis
    Rheumatoid arthritis
    Systemic sclerosis, telangiectasia syndrome
Genetically transmitted disease
    Rendu-Osler-Weber syndrome (hereditary hemorrhagic
        telangiectasia)
    Ataxia-telangiectasia
    Fabry's disease
    Xeroderma pigmentosum
States associated with prolonged vasodilatation (e.g., vari-
        cose veins, rosacea, polycythemia vera)
Peripheral vascular disease (e.g., livedo reticularis, erythema
        ab igne)
Neoplastic disease, especially
    Breast cancer
    Bile duct carcinoma
    Carcinoid tumor
    Cutaneous T-cell lymphoma
    Malignant angioendotheliomatosis
Radiation dermatitis
Mastocytosis

References

1. See Bibliography, 1.
2. See Bibliography, 3.

9-J. Urticaria

Specific antigen sensitivity (e.g., foods, food additives,
        Hymenoptera venom)
Physical agents
    Pressure, mechanical irritation, vibratory, water (aquagenic)
    Cold
    Heat
    Light (e.g., sunlight)
    Cholinergic urticaria
Atopic conditions (e.g., allergic rhinitis, asthma)
Drugs
    Opiates, barbiturates
    Antibiotics (especially penicillin, sulfonamides)
    X-ray contrast media

    NSAIDS, aspirin
    Thiazides
    Angiotensin-converting enzyme inhibitors
    D-Tubocurarine
    Azo dyes
    Quinine
    Curare
Transfusion of blood or blood components
Infections
    Bacterial (*Campylobacter enteritis*)
    Fungal (candidiasis)
    Viral (Hepatitis B, infectious mono, Coxsackie)
    Protozoal, helminths
Vasculitis
    Lupus erythematosus
    Rheumatoid arthritis
    Sjögren's syndrome
    Serum sickness
    Hepatitis B, acute
    Cryoglobulinemia
Mastocytosis (urticaria pigmentosa)
Occult malignancy (especially lymphoma, carcinoma)
Contact urticaria
    Plants (nettles)
    Animals
    Ammonium persulfate (hair bleaches)
Pregnancy, premenstrual
Angioedema (hereditary and acquired)
Emotional stress
Idiopathic

References

1. Bolognia JL, Braverman IM: Skin Manifestations of Internal Disease, p. 322. See Bibliography, 1.
2. Austen KF: Diseases of Immediate Type Hypersensitivity, pp. 1864–1868. See Bibliography, 1.
3. Habif TD: Clinical Dermatology, pp. 735–737. St. Louis: Mosby, 1996.

9-K. Vesicles and Bullae, Generalized*

Physical agents
    Radiation
    Burns

Chemicals
Cosmetics
Mechanical irritation, trauma
Metals (nickel, chromate)
Plants (poison ivy and oak, primrose)
Resins
Drugs
Barbiturates
Penicillins
Sulfonamides
Nitrofurantoin
Nalidixic acid
Bacitracin
Neomycin
Benzocaine
Thiazides
Furosemide
NSAIDs
Phenytoin
Mephenytoin
Allopurinol
Phenolphthalein
Infections
Bacterial
Disseminated gonococcus, *Pseudomonas*
Impetigo, erysipelas
Toxic epidermal necrolysis
Staphylococcal scalded skin syndrome
Viral
Herpes simplex
Herpes zoster
Varicella
Variola (smallpox)
Vaccinia
Enterovirus (e.g., hand-foot-mouth disease)
Syphilis, congenital
Rickettsialpox
Erythema multiforme bullosum, Stevens-Johnson syndrome
(see 9-B)
Pemphigus (vulgaris, foliaceus, erythematosus, paraneoplastic)
Pemphigoid (bullous, cicatricial)
Acute eczematous dermatitis, especially contact dermatitis
Dermatitis herpetiformis
Epidermolysis bullosa
Porphyria
Lupus erythematosus, discoid or systemic

Pityriasis rosea (vesicular type)
Diabetes mellitus
Herpes gestationis
Subcorneal pustular dermatosis
Bullous ichthyosis
Bullous insect bite eruption
Kaposi's varioliform eruption
Linear immunoglobulin A disease

References
1. Helm, pp. 162–177. See Bibliography, 2.
2. See Bibliography, 1.

*Vesicles are <0.5 cm and bullae are >0.5 cm.

9-L. Hypopigmentation

Vitiligo
    Diabetes
    Thyroid disease (thyroiditis)
    Pernicious anemia
    Collagen vascular diseases
Chemicals (monobenzyl ether of hydroquinone, mercury)
Congenital
Chemical leukoderma
Piebaldism
Nevus depigmentosus
Postinflammatory hypomelanosis
Tinea versicolor
Oculocutaneous albinism
Scleroderma
Tuberous sclerosis
Sarcoidosis
Cutaneous T-cell lymphoma
Vogt-Kayanagi-Harada syndrome
Psoriasis
Secondary syphilis

References
1. Johnson, pp. 187–194. See Bibliography, 6.
2. Fauci, pp. 316–317. See Bibliography, 1.
3. Sauer, pp. 253–255. See Bibliography, 3.

Bibliography

1. Fauci AS, Braunwald E, Isselbacher KJ, et al. (eds): *Harrison's Principles of Internal Medicine*, 14/e. New York: McGraw-Hill, 1997.
2. Helm KF, Marks JG: *Atlas of Differential Diagnosis in Dermatology*. New York: Churchill Livingstone, 1998.
3. Sauer GC, Hall JC: *Manual of Skin Diseases*. Philadelphia: Lippincott–Raven, 1996.
4. Habif TP: *Clinical Dermatology*. St. Louis: Mosby, 1996, p. 748.
5. Goldsmith LA, et al: *Adult and Pediatric Dermatology*. Philadelphia: FA Davis Co, 1997.
6. Johnson BL: *Ethnic Skin, Medical and Surgical*. St. Louis: Mosby, 1998, pp. 187–194.

10
MUSCULOSKELETAL SYSTEM

10-A. Shoulder Pain

Fracture
Contusion
Acromial-clavicular joint separation or injuries
Rotator cuff tendinitis or impingement syndrome
Bursitis
Bicipital tendinitis (long head)
Referred pain
    Diaphragmatic irritation
        Biliary disease
        Myocardial infarction
        Blood or gas in peritoneal or pleural cavity
        Subphrenic abscess
        Splenic trauma
        Neoplasm
        Lower lobe pleuropulmonary inflammatory disease
    Apical lung cancer (Pancoast's syndrome)
    Cervical radiculopathy and brachial neuritis
    Angina pectoris or myocardial infarction, or both
Osteoarthritis
Infectious arthritis
Rheumatoid arthritis
Crystalline arthritis
Arthritis associated with collagen-vascular disease
Rupture of rotator cuff
Anterior and posterior shoulder instability
Shoulder-hand syndrome

Neoplasm, primary or metastatic
Local arterial, venous, or lymphatic occlusion
Adhesive capsulitis
Thoracic outlet syndromes
    Cervical and first-rib syndromes, scalenus anterior
        syndrome
    Hyperabduction syndrome
    Costoclavicular syndrome
Myalgias and arthralgias fibrositis syndromes
Psychogenic pain
Sleep dysesthesias
Congenital or developmental abnormalities
Postural

References

1. Thornhill T: The Painful Shoulder, p. 491. See
   Bibliography, 1.
2. Canoso, pp. 238–253. See Bibliography, 3.
3. Neviaser RJ (ed): Management of Shoulder Problems.
   Orthop Clin North Am 18(3):373–444, 1987.

10-B. Back Pain

Functional, mechanical causes: postural imbalance
    Anteroposterior (e.g., pregnancy)
    Lateral (e.g., scoliosis, unequal leg lengths)
Trauma
    Lumbar strain or sprain
    Lumbosacral disc herniation
    Vertebral fracture (compression or other)
    Subluxation of facet joints
Osteoarthritis, spondylosis
Rheumatoid arthritis
Fibromyalgia
Polymyalgia rheumatica
Spondylitis or sacroiliitis, or both
    Ankylosing spondylitis
    Colitic (enteropathic) spondylitis
    Psoriatic arthritis
    Behçet's syndrome
    Reiter's syndrome
    Familial Mediterranean fever
    Syphilis

Ochronosis
Spinal stenosis
   Congenital
   Degenerative
   Iatrogenic (postlaminectomy, postfusion, or postchemo-
        nucleolysis)
   Post-traumatic
   Paget's disease
   Renal osteodystrophy
Spinal or vertebral tumor
   Benign (e.g., hemangioma, meningioma, osteoid osteoma)
   Malignant
      Primary (e.g., multiple myeloma, ependymoma,
           osteogenic sarcoma)
      Metastatic, especially
         Prostate
         Non-Hodgkin's lymphoma, Hodgkin's lymphoma
         Breast
         Leukemic
         Lung
         Kidney
         Thyroid
         Gastrointestinal tract
Infection (e.g., disc space infection, vertebral osteomyelitis,
        epidural abscess)
   Bacteria (usually secondary to hematogenous spread)
   Brucella
   Spirochetes
   Parasites
   Herpes zoster
   Mycobacteria
   Fungi
Congenital causes
   Facet hypertrophy
   Transitional vertebrae
   Spina bifida
   Spondylolysis, spondylolisthesis
Hyperparathyroidism
Osteomalacia (e.g., vitamin D–resistant rickets)
Osteoporosis (primary, endocrine, nutritional, drug)
Scheuermann's disease (epiphysitis)
Radium poisoning
Osteogenesis imperfecta
Referred pain
   Vascular disease (especially abdominal aortic aneurysm,
        Leriche's syndrome)

Hip pain
Pelvic or prostatic inflammation or tumor, endometriosis
Retroperitoneal hematoma or tumor
Renal disease
   Stone
   Infection
   Tumor
   Polycystic kidney disease
Abdominal disease (e.g., intestinal, pancreatic, gallbladder)
Cardiorespiratory (pulmonary emboli, pleuritis, coronary
     ischemia, pneumonitis)
Hematologic disorders
   Hemoglobinopathies (e.g., sickle cell, myelofibrosis)
Psychoneurotic causes
   Hysteria
   Malingering

References

1. Engstram J, Bradford D: Back and Neck Pain, pp. 73–79.
   See Bibliography, 1.
2. Wiesel S, et al: The Current Approach to the Medical
   Diagnosis of Low Back Pain. *Orthop Clin North Am*
   22(2):315, 1991.

10-C. Myalgias

Fibrositis
Connective tissue disease
   Polymyalgia rheumatica
   Rheumatoid arthritis
   Polymyositis, dermatomyositis
   Lupus erythematosus
   Polyarteritis nodosa
   Scleroderma
Systemic infection, especially
   Viral illness
      Influenza
      Coxsackievirus infection
      Human immunodeficiency virus (HIV)
      Dengue fever
      Arbovirus infection
      Hepatitis
      Rabies
      Poliomyelitis

Rheumatic fever
Salmonellosis
Tularemia
Brucellosis
Glanders
Trichinosis
Leptospirosis
Typhoid fever
Campylobacter
Malaria
Rhabdomyolysis (see 10-D)
Drugs (e.g., amphotericin B, clofibrate, carbenoxolone, chloroquine, cimetidine, glucocorticoids, zidovudine, oral contraceptives)
Hypothyroidism
Hyperparathyroidism
Hypoglycemic myopathy
Congenital enzyme deficiency [e.g., phosphorylase, (McArdle's disease), phosphofructokinase]
Polyneuropathy (e.g., Guillain-Barré disease)
Ischemic atherosclerotic disease (i.e., intermittent claudication)

Reference
1. Fauci, pp. 120, 429, 1136, 1844. See Bibliography, 1.

10-D. Muscle Weakness

Acute or Subacute*
Electrolyte abnormality
  Hyperkalemia
  Hypokalemia
  Hypercalcemia
  Hypermagnesemia
  Hypophosphatemia
Rhabdomyolysis
  Extreme muscular exertion
  Prolonged seizures
  Hyperthermia
  Extensive crush injury or muscle infarction
  Influenza
  Hypokalemia
  Hypophosphatemia
  Alcoholic myopathy
  Snake venoms

Industrial toxin ingestion
Familial myoglobinuria
Metabolic myopathies (e.g., McArdle's disease)
Polymyositis, dermatomyositis
Infection, especially
Viral
Influenza
Coxsackievirus infection
Rabies
Poliomyelitis
Herpes zoster
Trichinosis
Toxoplasmosis
Botulism
Diphtheria
Leprosy
Cysticercosis
Schistosomiasis
Trypanosomiasis
Landry-Guillain-Barré-Strohl syndrome
Peripheral neuropathy, acute (see 11-P)
Thyrotoxicosis
Corticosteroid therapy
Organophosphorous poisoning

Chronic
Progressive muscular dystrophies, especially
Oculopharyngeal
Duchenne's
Facioscapulohumeral
Limb-girdle
Myotonic
Endocrine disorders
Hyperthyroidism or hypothyroidism
Hyperparathyroidism
Vitamin D deficiency (e.g., vitamin D–deficiency rickets)
Corticosteroid therapy
Cushing's syndrome and Addison's disease
Acromegaly
Connective-tissue disease
Lupus erythematosus
Rheumatoid arthritis
Polymyositis, dermatomyositis
Sjögren's syndrome
Mixed connective tissue disease
Alcoholic myopathy

Chronic polymyopathy
  Glycogen storage diseases (e.g., McArdle's disease)
  Central core disease
Mitochondrial myopathy
  Lipid metabolism disorders (e.g., carnitine deficiency)
  Familial periodic paralysis with progressive myopathy
Progressive neural-muscular atrophy
  Amyotrophic lateral sclerosis
  Multiple sclerosis
  Werdnig-Hoffman disease
  Peroneal muscular atrophy (Charcot-Marie-Tooth disease)
  Chronic peripheral neuropathy (e.g., arsenic, lead, nutritional) (see 11-P)

Intermittent or Transient, or Both
Electrolyte abnormality
  Hypokalemia
  Hyperkalemia
  Hypophosphatemia
  Hypercalcemia
  Hypermagnesemia
  Hyperkalemic or (sodium channel disorders)
  Hypokalemic periodic paralysis (calcium channel disorders)
Drugs
  Aminoglycosides (especially neomycin, streptomycin, kanamycin, polymyxin B)
  Steroids
  Vincristine, zidovudine, cyclosporin
  Chloroquine
  Bretylium
  Clofibrate, pravastatin, gemfibrozil, niacin, lovastatin
Myasthenia gravis
Eaton-Lambert syndrome
Acute thyrotoxic myopathy
Thyrotoxic periodic paralysis
Paramyotonia congenita
Adynamia episodica hereditaria

References
1. Mendell J, Griggs R, Ptacek L: Diseases of Nerve and Muscle, pp. 2473–2483. See Bibliography, 1.
2. Miller M, Phelps P: Weakness, p. 388. See Bibliography, 2.

*Developing over days to weeks. (See Intermittent or Transient, or Both section)

10-E. Polyarticular Arthritis

Rheumatoid arthritis*
Juvenile rheumatoid arthritis*
Rheumatic fever*
Ankylosing spondylitis*
Collagen-vascular diseases
    Lupus erythematosus*
    Scleroderma*
    Polymyositis, dermatomyositis*
    Mixed connective tissue disease
    Polyarteritis nodosa (rare)*
    Henoch-Schönlein purpura (rare)*
    Wegener's granulomatosis (rare)*
    Other vasculitides (rare; e.g., allergic granulomatosis)*
    Polymyalgia rheumatica*
Immunologically mediated diseases
    Serum sickness*
    Hyperglobulinemic purpura*
    Hypogammaglobulinemia*
    Alpha-interferon induced
    Mixed cryoglobulinemia (rare)*
Systemic diseases
    Sjögren's syndrome*
    Reiter's syndrome*
    Psoriasis*
    Behçet's syndrome*
    Inflammatory bowel disease*
        Ulcerative colitis
        Regional enteritis
    Intestinal bypass*
    Pancreatic disease
        Carcinoma
        Pancreatitis
    Whipple's disease*
    Familial Mediterranean fever*
    Amyloidosis
    Sarcoidosis*
    Hematologic disorders
        Leukemia*
        Lymphoma*
        Multiple myeloma*
        Hemophilia
        Hemoglobinopathies (especially sickle cell anemia,
           thalassemia)*

Storage diseases (e.g., Gaucher's disease, Fabry's disease, hyperlipoproteinemia)*
- Ochronosis
- Hemochromatosis
- Wilson's disease
- Acromegaly
- Hypothyroidism
- Renal transplantation

Degenerative joint disease

Trauma

Neuropathic arthropathy (e.g., tabes dorsalis, diabetes mellitus, syringomyelia)

Joint tumor
- Pigmented villonodular synovitis
- Hemangioma
- Sarcoma

Infection*
- Bacterial (especially gonococcus, staphylococcus, pneumococcus)
- Viral (especially hepatitis B, mumps, rubella, arboviruses, parvovirus, retrovirus)
- Tuberculous
- Fungal (candida with central venous line or hyperalimentation)
- Rickettsial
- Parasitic
- Lyme disease

Others
- Gout*
- Pseudogout*
- Hypertrophic osteoarthropathy
- Intermittent hydrarthrosis*
- Palindromic rheumatism*
- Radiation
- Relapsing polychondritis*
- Acute tropical polyarthritis*
- Tietze's syndrome

Nonarticular rheumatism
- Bursitis*
- Periarthritis*
- Tendinitis*
- Tenosynovitis*
- Epicondylitis
- Myositis
- Fibrositis
- Fasciitis

References
1. See Bibliography, 2.
2. Nesher G, Ruchlemer : Alpha-Interferon–Induced Arthritis.
   Semin Arthritis Rheum 27(6):360–365, 1998.

*Usually inflammatory (i.e., joints painful, swollen, stiff, often erythematous and warm).

10-F. Monoarticular (Oligoarticular) Arthritis

Juvenile rheumatoid arthritis
Ankylosing spondylitis
Rheumatoid arthritis (rare)
Systemic diseases
    Psoriasis
    Behçet's syndrome
    Inflammatory bowel disease (ulcerative colitis, regional
           enteritis)
    Pancreatic disease (carcinoma, pancreatitis)
    Whipple's disease
    Familial Mediterranean fever
    Hematologic disorders
        Leukemia
        Lymphoma
        Bleeding-clotting disorders (hemophilia, von
            Willebrand's disease, anticoagulant use)
        Hemoglobinopathies (especially sickle cell anemia,
            thalassemia)
    Storage diseases (e.g., Gaucher's, Fabry's)
    Acromegaly
    Amyloidosis
Degenerative joint disease
Trauma
Neuropathic arthropathy (e.g., tabes dorsalis, diabetes melli-
        tus, syringomyelia)
Joint tumors (e.g., pigmented villonodular synovitis, heman-
        gioma, sarcoma)
Infection
    Bacterial (especially gonococcus, staphylococcus, pneu-
        mococcus)
    Viral (especially hepatitis B, rubella, mumps)
    Tuberculous
    Fungal
    Rickettsial
    Parasitic

Others
    Gout
    Pseudogout
    Intermittent hydrarthrosis
    Loose joint body
    Foreign body
    Palindromic rheumatism
    Radiation
    Relapsing polychondritis
Nonarticular rheumatism
    Bursitis
    Periarthritis
    Tendinitis
    Tenosynovitis
    Epicondylitis
    Myositis
    Fibrositis
    Fasciitis

Reference

1. McCune WJ: Monoarticular Arthritis, p. 371. See
   Bibliography, 2.

10-G. Characteristics of Synovial Fluid

	Normal	Noninflammatory	Inflammatory	Purulent	Hemorrhagic
Color	Clear to pale yellow	Xanthochromic	Xanthochromic to white	White	—
Clarity	Transparent	Transparent	Translucent to opaque	Opaque	—
Viscosity	High	High	Low	Low*	—
Mucin clot	Good	Good to fair	Fair to poor	Poor	—
Spontaneous clot	None	Often	Often	Often	—
WBCs/mm³	<150	<3,000	3,000–50,000	>50,000	—
% Polymorphs	<25	<25	>70	>90	—
Glucose (mg/dL)	Nearly equal to blood	Nearly equal to blood	>25, lower than blood	>50, lower than blood	—
Culture	Negative	Negative	Negative	Often positive	—
Conditions in which findings are likely to occur	—	Osteoarthritis Trauma Neuropathic arthropathy Chronic or subacute crystal synovitis	Rheumatoid arthritis Connective tissue diseases (SLE, PSS, DM/PM) Viral arthritis	Bacterial arthritis Tuberculous arthritis	Trauma Anticoagulation Neuropathic arthropathy: Charcot joints

SLE	Ankylosing spondylitis	Joint tumor (pigmented villonodular synovitis or hemangioma)
Scleroderma	Seronegative spondyloar-thropathies (Reiter's syndrome, psoriatic arthritis, inflammatory bowel disease arthritis)	Hematologic disorders (especially hemophilia, sickle cell trait or disease)
Polymyalgia rheumatica	Acute gout or pseudogout	Joint prosthesis
Erythema nodosum	Rheumatic fever	
Polyarteritis nodosa	Behçet's syndrome	
Amyloidosis		

DM/PM, dermatomyositis/polymyositis; PSS, progressive systemic sclerosis; SLE, systemic lupus erythematosus; WBCs, white blood cells.

*May be high in infection with coagulase-positive staphylococcus.

Group designations from Ropes MW, Bauer W: *Synovial Fluid Changes in Joint Diseases*. Cambridge, MA: Harvard University Press, 1953. Table modified from McCarty DJ, McCarty WJ (eds): *Arthritis and Allied Conditions*, 12/e. Philadelphia: Lea & Febiger, 1993:64–65; and from Schumacher HR (ed): *Primer on Rheumatic Diseases*, 9/e. Atlanta: Arthritis Foundation, 1988:55–60.

10-H. Clubbing

Usually with Hypertrophic Osteoarthropathy
Neoplasm
    Intrathoracic
        Lung
        Pleura
        Mediastinum (Hodgkin's disease)
        Thymus
    Esophagus, stomach
    Intestine
    Liver
Other pulmonary disorders
    Lung abscess
    Empyema
    Chronic interstitial pneumonitis
    Pneumoconiosis
    Sarcoidosis
    Bronchiectasis
    Tuberculosis
    Cystic fibrosis
Idiopathic, hereditary (pachydermoperiostosis)

Usually without Hypertrophic Osteoarthropathy
Genetic
Subacute bacterial endocarditis
Cyanotic congenital heart disease
Chronic liver disease (e.g., biliary cirrhosis)
Intestinal disorders
    Ulcerative colitis
    Regional enteritis
    Sprue, steatorrhea
    Bacterial or amebic dysentery
    Tuberculosis, intestinal
Hyperparathyroidism
Graves' disease (thyroid acropachy)
Occupational trauma (e.g., jackhammer operation)

Unilateral
Aneurysm of aorta or of subclavian, innominate, or
              brachial artery
Shoulder subluxation
Hemiplegia
Axillary or apical lung tumor

Unidigital
Median nerve injury
Sarcoidosis
Tophaceous gout

Reference
1. Altman RD, Tenenbaum J: Hypertrophic Osteoarthropathy, pp. 1514–1520. See Bibliography, 2.

10-I. Raynaud's Phenomenon

Raynaud's disease
Chronic arterial disease
    Atherosclerosis
    Thromboangiitis obliterans
    Thrombosis
    Embolism
Pulmonary veno-occlusive disease or primary pulmonary
        hypertension
Collagen-vascular disease
    Scleroderma
    Lupus erythematosus
    Rheumatoid arthritis
    Polyarteritis nodosa
    Mixed connective tissue disease
    Polymyositis, dermatomyositis
    Sjögren's syndrome
Occupational exposure
    Vibration (e.g., pneumatic tools)
    Percussion (e.g., typing)
    Vinyl chloride polymerization
Drugs, toxins
    Heavy metals (lead, arsenic, thallium)
    Methysergide, ergot compounds
    Beta-adrenergic blockers
    Chemotherapy (bleomycin, vinblastine, cisplatin)
Hematologic disorders
    Dysproteinemias (e.g., multiple myeloma, Waldenström's
        macroglobulinemia)
    Polycythemia vera, essential thrombocythemia
    Leukemia
    Cryoglobulinemia
    Cold agglutinin phenomenon

Neurologic disorders
    Peripheral neuropathy
    Hemiplegia
    Intervertebral disc herniation
    Spinal cord tumor
    Multiple sclerosis
    Transverse myelitis
    Syringomyelia
Carpal tunnel syndrome
Thoracic outlet syndrome
Post-traumatic reflex sympathetic dystrophy
Postcold injury (e.g., frostbite)
Acromegaly
Myxedema
Fabry's disease

References

1. Fauci, pp. 1401–1402. See Bibliography, 1.
2. Seibold JR: Scleroderma, p. 1133. See Bibliography, 1.

10-J. Osteomalacia

Vitamin D deficiency
    Dietary deficiency
    Insufficient sun exposure
    Malabsorption (e.g., pancreatic insufficiency, small-
        intestine disease, postgastrectomy)
Disordered vitamin D metabolism (hereditary or acquired)
    Chronic renal failure
    Anticonvulsant therapy
    Chronic liver disease (e.g., biliary cirrhosis)
Peripheral resistance to vitamin D (e.g., vitamin D–depend-
        ent rickets)
Chronic acidosis (e.g., distal renal tubular acidosis, chronic
        acetazolamide ingestion, ureterosigmoidostomy)
Phosphate depletion
Impaired renal tubular phosphate resorption
    Familial X-linked hypophosphatemia
    Fanconi syndrome (hereditary or acquired)
    Tumor phosphaturia
    Neurofibromatosis
    Neonatal (transient)

Intoxications (cadmium, lead, outdated tetracycline,
    aluminum)
Miscellaneous
    Osteopetrosis
    Hypophosphatasia
    Fluorosis
    Magnesium-dependent conditions
    Parenteral hyperalimentation
    Renal transplantation
    Tumor-associated renal disease
    Calcium deficiency due to biophosphonates

References
1. Raisy LG: Metabolic Bone Disease, p. 1228. See
   Bibliography, 4.
2. Krane SM, Holick MF: Metabolic Bone Disease, p. 2253.
   See Bibliography, 1.

10-K. Osteoporosis*

Aging (especially postmenopause)
Immobilization
Nutritional causes
    Calcium or vitamin D deficiency, or both
    Malnutrition, malabsorption
    Postgastrectomy
    Scurvy
    Total parenteral nutrition
    Pregnancy and lactation
    Aluminum-containing antacids
Corticosteroid excess
    Cushing's syndrome or disease
    Steroid therapy
Other endocrine disorders
    Hypogonadism (e.g., Klinefelter's syndrome, Turner's syn-
        drome, early oophorectomy)
    Thyrotoxicosis
    Acromegaly
    Hyperparathyroidism
    Hypopituitarism
    Diabetes mellitus
Inherited bone matrix abnormalities

Homocystinuria
Marfan's syndrome
Ehlers-Danlos syndrome
Osteogenesis imperfecta
Menkes' syndrome
Rheumatoid arthritis
Ankylosing spondylitis
Malignancy, especially
Lymphoma
Leukemia
Multiple myeloma
Waldenström's macroglobulinemia
Systemic mastocytosis
Carcinomatosis
Heparin therapy (chronic)
Chronic obstructive pulmonary disease
Chronic acidosis (especially renal tubular acidosis, metabolic
acidosis secondary to high-protein diet)
Alcoholism
Hepatic insufficiency, cirrhosis (alcoholic or other)
Methotrexate
Chronic anticonvulsant therapy
Chronic renal failure (renal osteodystrophy)
Paget's disease (with predominantly lytic lesions)
Juvenile (idiopathic)
Cystic fibrosis
Riley-Day syndrome
Menkes' syndrome
Down syndrome
Hypophosphatasia, adult variety
Female distance runners
Smoking

References

1. Raisy LG, et al: Metabolic Bone Disease. Endo 1998, p. 1225. See Bibliography, 4.
2. See Bibliography, 5.
3. Eastell R: Treatment of Postmenopausal Osteoporosis. *N Engl J Med* 338(11):736–746, 1998.

*Low bone mass and micro architectural deterioration of bone tissue leading to enhanced bone fragility and increased fracture risk.

Source: Consensus Development Conference: Diagnosis, Prophylaxis, and Treatment of Osteoporosis. *Am J Med* 94:636–638, 1993.

10-L. Antibodies to Nuclear or Cytoplamic Antigens

Disease	Antibodies most commonly associated
Systemic lupus erythematosus	Antinative (double-stranded) DNA Anti–single-stranded DNA Anti-Z-DNA Anti-histone (especially drug-induced lupus) Anti-Ku Anti-ribonucleoproteins (anti-snRNP; e.g. anti-SM) Anti-Ro/SS-A Anti-LA/SS-B Anti-RNA-polymerase (anti-RNAP)
Progressive systemic sclerosis	Anti-kinetochore (centromere) Anti-topoisomerase I (Scl-70) Anti-RNA-polymerase (anti-RNAP) Anti-RNP
Polymyositis/ scleroderma overlap syndrome	Myositis-specific autoantibodies (MSAs) Anti-tRNA-synthetases (anti-Jo, PL-7, PL-12, EJ, OJ) Anti-Mi-2 Anti-SnRNP Anti-PM-Sci
Mixed connective tissue disease	Anti-RNP (anti-UI snRNP)
Sjögren's syndrome	Anti-Ro/SS-A Anti-La/SS-B

References
1. Peng SL, Hardin JA, Craft J: Antinuclear Antibodies, pp. 250–265. See Bibliography, 2.
2. Schumacher HR (ed): *Primer on Rheumatic Diseases*, 9/e. Atlanta: Arthritis Foundation, 1988:35.
3. Reichlin M: Significance of Ro Antigen System. *J Clin Immunol* 6(5):339, 1986.

10-M. Rheumatoid Factor

Aging
Rheumatoid arthritis
Systemic lupus erythematosus

Progressive systemic sclerosis
Dermatomyositis, polymyositis
Infections
    Syphilis
    Influenza
    Subacute bacterial endocarditis
    Infectious mononucleosis
    Bacterial bronchitis
    Viral hepatitis
    Tuberculosis
    Leprosy
    Parasitic infection (e.g., schistosomiasis, kala-azar)
    After extensive immunizations
    Lyme disease
    Acquired immunodeficiency syndrome (AIDS)
    Cytomegalovirus
    Rubella
    Periodontal disease
Sjögren's syndrome (with or without arthritis)
Chronic active hepatitis and cirrhosis
Lymphoma
Waldenström's macroglobulinemia
Mixed cryoglobulinemia
Hypergammaglobulinemic purpura
Chronic lung disease
    Pneumoconiosis (e.g., silicosis, asbestosis)
    Sarcoidosis
    Interstitial fibrosis, idiopathic
Multiple transfusions
Renal transplantation

References
1. Lipsky PE: Rheumatoid Arthritis, p. 1437. See Bibliography, 1.
2. Koopman, p. 1121. See Bibliography, 6.

10-N. Systemic Lupus Erythematosus Criteria*

Facial erythema (butterfly rash)
Discoid lupus erythematosus
Photosensitivity
Nonerosive arthritis
Oral or nasopharyngeal ulceration
Serositis (pleuritis or pericarditis, or both)

Psychosis or seizures, or both
Proteinuria >0.5 g/day or cellular casts in urine (red cell,
hemoglobin, granular, tubular, mixed)
Hematologic disorder
Hemolytic anemia, leukopenia (WBC <4,000/mm^3), lym-
phopenia (<1,500/mm^3), or thrombocytopenia
(<100,000/mm^3)
Antinuclear antibody
Immunologic disorder: positive lupus erythematosus cell
preparation, anti-DNA antibodies, anti-Sm antibodies, or chronic false-positive serologic test for
syphilis

*Diagnosis of systemic lupus can be made if of the 11 criteria are
present, serially or simultaneously, during any interval of observation.

Source: Tan EM, et al: The 1982 Revised Criteria for the Classification of
Systemic Lupus Erythematosus (SLE). *Arthritis Rheum* 25:1271, 1982.

Bibliography

1. Fauci AS, et al: *Harrison's Principles of Internal
   Medicine*, 14/e. New York: McGraw-Hill, 1998.
2. Kelly WN, et al: *Textbook of Rheumatology*, 5/e.
   Philadelphia: WB Saunders, 1997.
3. Canoso J: *Rheumatology in Primary Care*. Philadelphia:
   WB Saunders, 1997.
4. Wilson J, Foster D, Kronenberg H, Larsen PR: *Williams
   Textbook of Endocrinology*, 9/e. Philadelphia: WB
   Saunders, 1998.
5. Carey CF, Lee HL, Woeltje KF (eds): *The Washington
   Manual of Medical Therapeutics*, 29/e. Philadelphia:
   Lippincott–Raven, 1998.
6. Koopman WJ (ed): *Arthritis and Allied Conditions*, 12/e.
   Philadelphia: Lea & Febiger, 1997.
7. Fitzpatrick TB, et al. (eds): *Textbook of Rheumatology*,
   3/e. Philadelphia: WB Saunders, 1989.
8. Johnson BL: *Ethnic Skin, Medical and Surgical*. St.
   Louis: Mosby, 1998.
9. Wilson JD, et al. (eds): *Harrison's Principles of Internal
   Medicine*, 12/e. New York: McGraw-Hill, 1991.
10. Sauer GC, Hall JC: *Manual of Skin Diseases*.
    Philadelphia: Lippincott–Raven, 1996.

11 NERVOUS SYSTEM

11-A. Dizziness and Vertigo

Dizziness
Hyperventilation
Anxiety, psychosomatic causes
Hypoxia
Anemia
Visual disturbances
    Incorrect spectacles
    Sudden extraocular muscle paresthesia with diplopia
Hypotension (especially orthostatic)
Hypertension
Cardiac arrhythmia
Peripheral neuropathy
Myelopathy
Concussion
Aging
Syncope of any cause (see 11-D)

True Vertigo
Infection
    Labyrinthitis (bacterial, viral, syphilitic)
    Cholesteatoma
    Chronic otitis media with middle-ear fistula
    Vestibular neuronitis or neuropathy
    Herpes zoster oticus
Vascular disorders
    Vertebrobasilar insufficiency or occlusion

Vascular malformations
Labyrinthine or internal auditory artery occlusion or spasm
Migraine
Hemorrhage into labyrinthine system, brainstem, or cere-
  bellum (e.g., secondary to bleeding diathesis,
  leukemia, hypertension)
Ménière's disease
Benign positional vertigo of Bárány
Drugs and toxins
  Alcohol
  Quinine
  Ethacrynic acid
  Aminoglycoside antibiotics (especially streptomycin,
    gentamicin)
  Salicylates
  Benzene
  Arsenic
  Arsine
Trauma
  Temporal bone fracture
  Labyrinthine concussion
  Postsurgical (inner-ear area)
  Perilymphatic fistula
Tumor, especially
  Acoustic neuroma
  Epidermoid carcinoma
  Metastatic carcinoma (especially breast, kidney, lung,
    stomach)
  Glomus body tumor
Other
  Unusual head or neck positions
  Cerumen impaction
  Motion sickness
  Space sickness
  Multiple sclerosis
  Extraocular muscle palsy
  Syringobulbia
  Tabes dorsalis
  Friedreich's ataxia
  Encephalitis
  Seizure aura or temporal lobe seizure
  Psychogenic

References

1. Deafness, Dizziness, and Disorders of Equilibrium, p.
   747. See Bibliography, 1.

2. Wazen JJ: Dizziness and Hearing Loss in General, p. 30. See Bibliography, 2.
3. Longridge NS: Approach to the Patient with Dizziness and Vertigo, p. 2320. See Bibliography, 3.

11-B. Headache

Muscle contraction (tension)
Migraine
Cluster (histamine) headache
Nonmigrainous vascular causes
    Effort (physical activity)
    Vasomotor rhinitis
    Cough (e.g., Arnold-Chiari syndrome)
    Fever
    Hypertension
    Hypotension
    Hypoxia or hypercapnia, or both (e.g., chronic obstructive pulmonary disease, pulmonary infiltrative disease, sleep apnea syndrome, high altitude)
    Anemia
    Cerebrovascular disease (thrombosis, embolism, hemorrhage)
    Postseizure
    Post–lumbar puncture
    Endocrine causes
        Hypoglycemia
        Hypothyroidism
        Hyperthyroidism
        Adrenal insufficiency
        Carcinoid, serotonin-secreting tumors
        Premenstrual syndrome
        Polycystic ovary syndrome
Drugs and toxins
    Theophylline
    Caffeine and caffeine withdrawal
    Nitrates
    Nitrites (e.g., hot dogs)
    Dextroamphetamines
    Ephedrine
    Oral contraceptives
    Reserpine
    Monamine oxidase inhibitors plus catecholamines
    Monosodium glutamate (MSG)

Histamine
Steroid withdrawal
Alcohol withdrawal
Disulfiram (Antabuse) plus alcohol
Lead
Benzene
Carbon monoxide
Carbon tetrachloride
Insecticides
Intracranial causes
  Tumor
  Arteriovenous malformation
  Aneurysm (with or without hemorrhage)
  Subdural hematoma
  Encephalitis, brain abscess
  Pseudotumor cerebri
  Post-traumatic
  Other lesions (e.g., sarcoidosis)
  Arnold-Chiari malformation
  Cranial inflammation
    Meningeal irritation or inflammation
      Infection (e.g., bacterial, viral, tuberculous, fungal)
      Carcinomatous infiltration
      Intrathecal injection
    Postsubarachnoid hemorrhage
    Vasculitis (e.g., temporal arteritis, lupus, polyarteritis
      nodosa)
  Cranial and neck causes
    Cranial bone lesions
    Sinuses (trauma, inflammation)
    Ears (external, middle, internal)
    Eyes (inflammation, trauma, increased intraocular
      pressure, poor refraction)
    Teeth, jaws (infection, trauma, temporomandibular joint
      malocclusion)
    Cervical spine, ligaments, muscles (trauma, cervical
      spondylosis, ankylosing spondylitis, tumor)
    Neuralgia (e.g., postherpetic, trigeminal, glosso-
      pharyngeal)
Psychogenic, psychiatric
Systemic diseases
  Infectious mononucleosis
  Systemic lupus erythematosus
  Hashimoto's thyroiditis
  Inflammatory bowel disease
  Acquired immunodeficiency syndrome (AIDS)–related
    illnesses

References
1. Lance JW: Approach to the Patient with Headaches, p. 206. See Bibliography, 3.
2. Headache and Other Craniofacial Pain, p. 148. See Bibliography, 1.
3. Raskin NH: Headache, p. 42. See Bibliography, 2.

11-C. Paresthesias

Peripheral neuropathy (see 11-Q), especially associated with
    Diabetes mellitus
    Alcoholism
    Thiamine deficiency
Peripheral nerve entrapment, compression, trauma (e.g., intervertebral disc herniation, thoracic duct outlet syndrome, carpal tunnel syndrome)
Atherosclerotic peripheral vascular disease
Spinal cord disease
    Spinal cord or nerve root compression
    Multiple sclerosis
    Tabes dorsalis
    Subacute combined degeneration of spinal cord (pernicious anemia, vitamin B_{12} deficiency)
    Strachan's syndrome
Cortical or thalamic lesions
Metabolic disturbance
    Hypocalcemia
    Respiratory alkalosis

References
1. Other Somatic Sensations, p. 130. See Bibliography, 1.
2. Thompson HG, Rowland LP: Diagnosis of Pain and Paresthesia, p. 27. See Bibliography, 2.

11-D. Syncope

Neurologic or Mechanical Causes, or Both
Mediated by vagal stimulation or autonomic insufficiency, or both
    Vasovagal reaction (often associated with strong emotion or pain)

Prolonged recumbency or inactivity
Peripheral neuropathy with autonomic involvement (e.g.,
      diabetes, amyloidosis, tabes dorsalis) (see 11-Q)
Drugs (e.g., nitrates, antihypertensive agents, ganglionic
      blockers, alcohol)
Carotid sinus syncope
Micturition syncope
Swallow syncope
Stretch syncope
Bowel stimulation or defecation syncope
Airway stimulation (e.g., suctioning)
Eyeball pressure
Glossopharyngeal neuralgia
Syringomyelia
Shy-Drager syndrome
Sympathectomy
Primary autonomic insufficiency
Seizure
Head trauma
Reduced cardiac output or venous return
  Hypovolemia
  Hypotension
  Valsalva maneuver
    Cough
    Voluntary forced expiration against closed glottis
    Weight lifting
  Atrial myxoma or thrombus
  Cardiac tamponade

Cardiopulmonary Causes
Cardiac arrhythmias (see 2-O)
  Bradyarrhythmias (e.g., sick sinus syndrome)
  Tachyarrhythmias (especially ventricular fibrillation, ventric-
      ular tachycardia, paroxysmal atrial tachycardia)
  Atrioventricular block
Pulmonary embolism
Myocardial infarction with cardiogenic shock
Pericardial tamponade
Aortic stenosis
Pulmonic stenosis
Primary pulmonary hypertension
Congenital heart disease
Cardiomyopathies (see 2-H)
Shock (see 2-K)
Atrial myxoma or thrombus
Prosthetic valve thrombosis or obstruction

Cerebrovascular Causes
Atherosclerotic disease of carotid and/or cerebral vessels
(especially vertebral-basilar insufficiency)
Subclavian steal
Takayasu's arteritis
Hypertensive encephalopathy
Cervical spine abnormalities (e.g., cervical spondylosis)

Metabolic Causes
Anemia
Hypoxia
Hyperventilation
Hypoglycemia
Adrenal insufficiency

Psychological Causes
Anxiety, hysteria

References
1. Pedley TA, Ziegler DK: Syncope and Seizure, p. 12. See
   Bibliography, 2.
2. Friedman HH: Syncope, p. 395. See Bibliography, 4.

11-E. Deafness

Sensorineural (Inner Ear)
Aging
Prolonged exposure to loud noise
Drugs
    Salicylates
    Aminoglycoside antibiotics (especially neomycin, amikacin)
    Furosemide, ethacrynic acid
    Quinine
    Cisplatin
Infection
    Meningitis
    Chronic middle or inner ear infection
    Cholesteatoma
    Labyrinthitis
        Bacterial
        Viral (e.g., mumps)
        Syphilis (usually congenital)

Herpes zoster oticus
Autoimmune disease (e.g., polyarteritis nodosa, Cogan's
    syndrome)
Ménière's disease
Fractures of temporal bone
Cochlear otosclerosis
Tumor of eighth nerve or cerebellopontine angle (especially
    acoustic neuroma)
Eighth nerve infarction
Multiple sclerosis
Hereditary or congenital causes (e.g., congenital rubella,
    Alport's syndrome)
Any central auditory pathway lesion (e.g., small strokes, mul-
    tiple sclerosis)

Conductive
Cerumen impaction and foreign bodies
Otosclerosis
Chronic otitis media, cholesteatoma
Trauma (including temporal bone fracture, bleeding into
    middle ear)
Mucopolysaccharidoses
Neoplasm

References
1. Deafness, Dizziness, and Disorders of Equilibrium, p.
   247. See Bibliography, 1.
2. Wazen JJ: Dizziness and Hearing Loss, p. 80. See
   Bibliography, 2.

11-F. Ataxia

Symmetric and Progressive Cerebellar Signs
Acute (hours to days)
  Toxic
    Alcohol
    Lithium
    Phenytoin
    Barbiturates
    Carbamazepine
  Heatstroke
  Viral cerebellitis

Seizure disorder
Postinfection syndrome
Hypoglycemia
Hyponatremia
Hypoxic encephalopathy
Cranial trauma
Subacute (days to weeks)
Toxic
Arsenic-bismuth
Mercury
Lead
Glue and paint sniffing
Toluene exposure
Spray painting
Chemotherapeutics
Thallium
Organophosphates
Alcoholic nutritional (e.g., vitamin B_1 and B_2 deficiency)
Lyme disease
Miscellaneous infections (e.g., viral, toxoplasmosis)
Chronic (months to years)
Paraneoplastic syndrome
Hypothyroidism
Tabes dorsalis
Inherited ataxias
Meningovascular syphilis
Vitamin E deficiency

Focal and Ipsilateral Cerebellar Signs
Acute (hours to days)
Vascular
Cerebellar hemorrhage
Subdural hematoma
Infarction
Vasculitis
Cerebellar abscess
Subacute (days to weeks)
Acute multiple sclerosis
Primary or metastatic neoplasm
AIDS–related progressive multifocal leukoencephalopathy
or lymphoma
Chronic (months to years)
Stable gliosis due to stroke or demyelinating plaque
Dandy-Walker or Arnold-Chiari malformations

References
1. Rosenberg RN: Ataxic Disorders, p. 2363. See
   Bibliography, 5.
2. Bressman SB: Ataxias, p. 686. See Bibliography, 2.

11-G. Acute Confusional State or Coma, or Both*

Usually No Lateralizing Signs, Normal Brainstem Reflexes
Drug withdrawal after chronic intoxication, especially
   Alcohol
   Barbiturates
   Other sedatives
Drug intoxication, especially
   Atropine
   Amphetamines
   Barbiturates and other neuroleptics
   Bromides
   Caffeine
   Carbon monoxide
   Corticosteroids
   Lithium
   Metoclopramide
   Narcotics
   Scopolamine
   Tricyclic antidepressants
Infectious illness, especially
   Septicemia
   Meningitis
   Pneumonia
   Typhoid fever
   Creutzfeldt-Jakob disease
   Rheumatic fever
   Progressive multifocal leukoencephalopathy
Central nervous system disorders
   Bilateral subdural hematoma
   Cerebrovascular disease (especially involving parietal or
            temporal lobes or upper brainstem)
   Viral encephalitis (nonherpetic)
   Subarachnoid hemorrhage
   Hydrocephalus
   Head trauma (e.g., concussion)
   Seizures and postictal state
   Fat embolism

Migraine
Carcinomatosis meningitis
Hysterical coma or catatonia
Metabolic causes
    Pancreatitis
    Hyperviscosity syndrome
    Adrenal insufficiency
    Hyponatremia or hypernatremia
    Hypocalcemia or hypercalcemia
    Hypomagnesemia or hypermagnesemia
    Hypophosphatemia or hyperphosphatemia
    Hypokalemia or hyperkalemia
    Hypoxia
    Hypercarbia
    Congestive heart failure and other hypoperfusion states
        (see 2-K)
    Hypoglycemia or hyperglycemia
    Hepatic encephalopathy
    Uremia
    Hypothyroidism or hyperthyroidism
    Wernicke's disease
    Porphyria
    Severe metabolic acidosis or alkalosis
    Severe hyperthermia or hypothermia
    Hypo-osmolality or hyperosmolality
    Hypertensive encephalopathy
    Reye's syndrome
    Febrile illness
    Acute psychosis (e.g., postoperative, postpartum)
    Preexisting dementia with superimposed stress
        (see 11-H)

***Usually with Lateralizing Signs, Normal
Brainstem Reflexes***
Intracerebral hemorrhage
Large cerebral infarction with edema
Herpesvirus encephalitis
Subdural or epidural hematoma or empyema
Tumor (especially with edema)
Brain abscess with edema
Vasculitis with infarction
Metabolic encephalopathy with preexisting focal lesion
Pituitary apoplexy
Thrombotic thrombocytopenic purpura (TTP)
Focal seizure or postictal state

Cerebellar or Brainstem Lesion
with Multiple Abnormal Reflexes
Hemorrhage
Neoplasm
Infarct
Contusion
Abscess
Demyelination
Encephalitis
Migraine of basilar artery
Severe drug overdose

*Modified from Wilson JD, et al. (eds): *Harrison's Principles of Internal Medicine*, 14/e. New York: McGraw-Hill, 1998, p. 133.

11-H. Dementia*

Degenerative diseases
   Alzheimer's disease
   Cerebral arteriosclerosis, multiple cerebrovascular
      accidents
   Pick's disease (frontal temporal dementia)
   Parkinson's disease
   Korsakoff's psychosis
   Demyelinating disease [e.g., multiple sclerosis, Schilder's
      disease (diffuse cerebral sclerosis)]
   Amyotrophic lateral sclerosis
   Progressive supranuclear palsy (Steele-Richardson-
      Olszewski syndrome)
Metabolic causes
   Hypoxic encephalopathy
   Hypoglycemia
   Hypocalcemia (e.g., hypoparathyroidism)
   Hepatocerebral degeneration (posthepatic coma)
   Pernicious anemia, subacute combined degeneration of
      the spinal cord
   Heavy metal intoxication
   Pellagra
   Myxedema
   Cushing's disease
   Chronic barbiturate intoxication
   Bromide intoxication
   Dialysis dementia
   Mitochondrial encephalopathies

Infectious causes
   Brain abscess
   Chronic meningoencephalitis (e.g., cryptococcosis,
         neurosyphilis)
   Viral encephalitis (especially herpes simplex)
   AIDS
   Progressive multifocal leukoencephalopathy
   Creutzfeldt-Jakob disease
Intracranial tumor
Head trauma (e.g., contusion, hemorrhage, subdural hematoma)
Vasculitis
Myoclonic epilepsy
Normal-pressure hydrocephalus
Hereditary diseases
   Huntington's chorea
   Wilson's disease
   Lipid storage diseases (e.g., Tay-Sachs, leukodystrophies)
   Mucopolysaccharidoses
Pseudodementias
   Depression
   Hypomania
   Schizophrenia
   Hysteria

References
1. Sacktor NC, Mayeux R: Delirium and Dementia, p. 1. See
   Bibliography, 2.
2. Miller BC: Chronic Dementing Conditions, p. 2390. See
   Bibliography, 3.

*Deterioration of intellectual and cognitive functions with little or no dis-
turbance of consciousness or perception.

11-I. Tremor

Tremor at rest (present at rest, decreased with movement)
   Parkinson's disease
   Postencephalitic parkinsonism
   Wilson's disease
   Phenothiazines (tardive dyskinesia)
   Metoclopramide
   Selective serotonin reuptake inhibitor (SSRI) antidepressants
   Brain tumor

Action tremor (present with movement, decreased at rest)
  Physiologic (anxiety, fatigue)
  Essential (senile or familial, or both)
  Cerebellar disease
  Withdrawal from alcohol or opiates
Orthostatic tremor
  Meningoencephalitis (e.g., viral, paretic neurosyphilis)
  Hyperthyroidism
  Fever
  Pheochromocytoma
  Hypoglycemia
  Parkinson's disease (rarely)
  Carcinoid syndrome
  Bronchodilators, β-agonists
  Xanthines (e.g., coffee, tea)
  Steroids
  Valproic acid
  Bromide and bismuth intoxications
  Lithium
Ataxic or intension tremor (increased at terminal phase of
          voluntary movement) (see 11-F)
  Cerebellar disease
  Multiple sclerosis
  Vascular midbrain and subthalamic lesions

References
1. Tremor, Myoclonus Spasms and Tics, p. 85. See
   Bibliography, 1.
2. Greene P: Essential Tremor, p. 712. See Bibliography, 2.

11-J. Choreoathetosis

Hereditary diseases, especially
  Wilson's disease
  Huntington's disease
  Neuroacanthocytosis
  Ataxia telangiectasia
  Lesch-Nyhan disease
  Lipid storage disease (e.g., Niemann-Pick)
  Dystonia musculorum deformans
  Hereditary nonprogressive chorea
Drugs
  Phenothiazines
  Haloperidol

L-Dopa
Dihydroxyphenylalanine
Bromocriptine
Anticholinergics
Postinfectious (Sydenham's chorea)
   Rheumatic fever
   Diphtheria
   Rubella
   Pertussis
Pregnancy (chorea gravidarum)
Estrogen therapy (e.g., oral contraceptives)
Multiple sclerosis
Hypoxic encephalopathy
Kernicterus
Senile chorea
Perinatal hypoxia or injury
Hypoparathyroidism
Hyperthyroidism
Non-Wilsonian hepatocerebral degeneration (posthepatic coma)
Lupus erythematosus
Periarteritis nodosa
Antiphospholipid syndrome
Acute disseminated encephalomyelitis (postinfectious, post-
         vaccinal)
Nonketotic hyperosmolar coma
Corticostriatospinal degeneration
Subthalamic infarct or hemorrhage (hemiballism)

Reference
1. Fahn S: Sydenham and Other Forms of Chorea, p. 699.
   See Bibliography, 2.

11-K. Nystagmus

Pendular*
Congenital
Spasmus nutans
Associated with bilateral central loss of vision before 2 years
         of age
   Albinism
   Aniridia
   Bilateral chorioretinitis
   Congenital cataracts
   Corneal scarring

Optic atrophy
Multiple sclerosis
Prolonged work in dim light (miner's nystagmus)

Jerk[†]
Nonpathologic
  Extreme lateral gaze
  Attempt to fix on moving objects (opticokinetic nystagmus)
  Labyrinthine stimulation (e.g., cold water in auditory canal)
Drugs
  Barbiturates
  Alcohol
  Phenytoin
  Haloperidol
  Phenothiazines
  Meperidine
  Lithium, thallium, and organophosphate intoxications
Labyrinthine-vestibular disease (e.g., aminoglycoside tox-
      icity) (see 11-A)
Cerebellar lesions (e.g., Wernicke's disease, cerebellopon-
      tine angle tumor)
Encephalitis
Severe magnesium deficiency
Vascular disease involving brainstem (especially hyperten-
      sive infarction, posterior-inferior cerebellar artery
      occlusion)
Demyelinating disease (e.g., multiple sclerosis)
Brainstem tumor and other lesions
Syringobulbia
Paraneoplastic syndromes
Meningioma, meningeal cyst
Arnold-Chiari malformation
Parinaud syndrome
Congenital

Reference
1. Disorders of Ocular Movement and Papillary Functions, p.
   237. See Bibliography, 1.

*Both components equal.
†Fast and slow components.

11-L. Seizures

Central Nervous System and Vascular Causes
Cerebrovascular disease (see 11-N)
  Thrombosis
  Embolism
  Hemorrhage (intracerebral or subarachnoid)
  Vasculitis (especially lupus erythematosus, polyarteritis
      nodosa, mixed connective tissue disease)
  Old infarction
  Thrombophlebitis
  Arteriovenous malformation
Brain tumor (especially metastatic tumor, meningioma, astro-
      cytoma)
Cerebral infection
  Encephalitis
  Meningitis (especially bacterial)
  Brain abscess
  Human immunodeficiency syndrome (HIV) encephalopathy
  Neurosyphilis
  Creutzfeldt-Jakob disease
Head trauma
Hypoxic encephalopathy
Reduced cerebral blood flow (e.g., hypotension, Stokes-
      Adams syndrome, carotid sinus syncope)
Hypertensive encephalopathy
Eclampsia
Alzheimer's disease
Pick's disease
Multiple sclerosis

Metabolic Causes
Fever
Alcohol withdrawal
Barbiturate withdrawal
Benzodiazepine or other sedative withdrawal
Drugs, toxins
  Amphetamines
  Heroin
  Cocaine
  Phencyclidine
  Methylphenidate
  Phenothiazines
  Tricyclic antidepressants

    Lidocaine
    Aminophylline
    Salicylates
    Ergot
    Digitalis
    Erythropoietin
    Bupropion
    Cyclosporin
    Penicillins and β-lactam antibiotics
    Quinolones
    Isoniazid
    Cycloserine
    Physostigmine, other anticholinergics
    Vincristine
    Lithium
    Lead
    Mercury
    Arsenic
    Thallium
    Strychnine
    Camphor
Hypoglycemia
Hyperglycemia
Hyponatremia
Hypernatremia (or rapid correction of hypernatremia)
Hypocalcemia
Hypomagnesemia
Alkalosis (respiratory or metabolic)
Uremia
Dialysis dysequilibrium
Hepatic failure
Reye's syndrome
Thyrotoxicosis
Hypothyroidism
Pyridoxine deficiency
Pellagra

Congenital or Inherited Diseases
Congenital infection
    Toxoplasmosis
    Cytomegalovirus
    Syphilis
    Rubella (maternal)
Neonatal hypoxia or trauma, kernicterus
Down syndrome

Lipid storage disease (e.g., Gaucher's disease)
Tuberous sclerosis
Sturge-Weber disease
Phenylketonuria
Acute intermittent porphyria
Argininosuccinicaciduria

Idiopathic Epilepsy
Generalized
    Tonic-clonic (grand mal)
    Absence (petit mal)
    Lennox-Gastaut syndrome
    Juvenile myoclonic epilepsy
    Infantile spasms (West's syndrome)
    Atonic
Partial or focal
    Simple (without loss of consciousness)
        Motor
        Somatosensory
        Autonomic
        Psychic
    Complex (with impaired consciousness)
Special epileptic syndromes
    Myoclonus
    Reflex epilepsy
    Acquired aphasia with convulsive disorder
    Hysterical

References
1. Pedley TA, Scheue ML, Walczak TS: Epilepsy, p. 845. See Bibliography, 2.
2. Epilepsy and Other Seizure Disorders, p. 273. See Bibliography, 1.

11-M. Cerebrovascular Disease

Thrombosis or Vascular Occlusion, or Both
Thrombosis, atherosclerotic
Hypotension in presence of atherosclerotic carotid disease
        (e.g., hypovolemia, Stokes-Adams attack, myocardial infarction)

Vasculitis (especially arteritis)
  Infectious
    Subacute bacterial meningitis
    Meningovascular syphilis
    Tuberculous meningitis
    Fungal meningitis
    Protozoan and parasitic meningitis (e.g., malaria, trichi-
        nosis, schistosomiasis)
    HIV–related
  Noninfectious
    Systemic lupus erythematosus
    Polyarteritis nodosa
    Sjögren's syndrome
    Necrotizing arteritis
    Granulomatous arteritis (e.g., Wegener's)
    Lymphomatoid granulomatosis
    Temporal arteritis
    Takayasu's disease
    Behçet's syndrome
Cerebral thrombophlebitis and/or venous sinus thrombosis
        (usually associated with infection of ear, sinus,
        face, or meninges)
Oral contraceptives
Hematologic disorders
  Sickle cell disease
  Factor C or S deficiency
  Polycythemia vera
  TTP
  Thrombocytosis
  Hyperproteinemic or hyperviscosity states
  Hypercoagulable state
  Antiphospholipid antibodies
  Diffuse intravascular coagulation
Carotid artery trauma
Radiation
Closed head trauma
Eclampsia
Postarteriographic
Cocaine, heroin, and amphetamine use
Dissecting aneurysm of carotid artery (e.g., secondary to
        cystic medial necrosis or dissecting aortic
        aneurysm)
Pressure secondary to intracerebral hematoma
Migraine syndrome
Fibromuscular dysplasia
Fabry's disease

Homocystinuria
Moyamoya disease
Binswanger's disease
Mitochondrial encephalopathy, lactic acidosis, and strokelike
episodes (MELAS)

Embolism
Atrial arrhythmias (especially atrial fibrillation—usually with
rheumatic valvular or atherosclerotic cardiovas-
cular disease)
Rheumatic and other valvular heart disease, especially mitral
stenosis (with or without atrial fibrillation)
Myocardial infarction with mural thrombus
Cardiac surgery, complications of (e.g., air, platelet, fat, sili-
cone embolism)
Prosthetic heart valve
Cardiomyopathy (see 2-H)
Endocarditis
Bacterial
Nonbacterial (e.g., associated with carcinomatosis or sys-
temic lupus erythematosus)
Congenital heart disease
Atherosclerotic embolism from other arteries
Aorta or carotid arteries (e.g., secondary to carotid mas-
sage or arteriography)
Vertebral or basilar arteries
Pulmonary vein thrombosis (especially septic or tumor emboli)
Fat embolism
Tumor embolism
Air embolism
Venous thromboembolism with cardiac or pulmonary right-to-
left shunt (paradoxic embolism)
Atrial myxoma
Trichinosis

Hemorrhage
Hypertension (including hypertensive encephalopathy)
Aneurysm (ruptured or unruptured)
Saccular ("berry")
Fusiform (atherosclerotic)
Mycotic
Arteriovenous malformation, ruptured or unruptured
Hemorrhagic disorders (e.g., thrombocytopenia, thrombocy-
tosis, coagulopathy, disseminated intravascular
coagulation, anticoagulant therapy)

Intracranial trauma (e.g., acute extradural or subdural
hematoma, intracerebral hemorrhage)
Hemorrhage into tumor
Hemorrhagic infarction
Connective-tissue disease (especially lupus erythematosus
and polyarteritis nodosa)

References
1. Cerebrovascular Disease, p. 669. See Bibliography, 1.
2. Yatsee PM: Other Cerebrovascular Syndromes, p. 257.
See Bibliography, 3.

11-N. Paralysis and Paresis

Acute (Developing in Hours)
Spinal cord injury
Spinal cord hemorrhage (secondary to vascular malforma-
tion, coagulopathy, anticoagulant therapy, trauma)
Spinal cord infarct (secondary to spinal artery thrombosis,
embolism, vasculitis)
Dissecting aortic aneurysm
Aortic thrombosis
Acute necrotizing myelitis
Profound hypokalemia (serum K^+ <2.5 mEq/L)
Hyperkalemic or hypokalemic periodic paralysis
Hypermagnesemia

Subacute (Developing in Days)
Guillain-Barré syndrome
Myelitis
Viral (especially polio, rabies, herpes zoster)
Postinfectious (especially after measles, smallpox, chick-
enpox)
Subacute pyogenic meningomyelitis
Tuberculous meningomyelitis
Acute demyelinating myelitis (e.g., multiple sclerosis)
Acute necrotizing myelitis
Rhabdomyolysis
Crush injury
Excessive muscular activity
Muscle infarction secondary to prolonged pressure and
ischemia

Polymyositis, viral or idiopathic
Diphtheritic polyneuropathy
Botulism
Spinal cord or epidural abscess
Spinal cord compression (e.g., secondary to tumor)

Slow (Developing over Weeks to Months)
Severe peripheral neuropathy (see 11-Q)
Multiple cerebrovascular accidents (bilateral hemiplegia)
Polymyositis
    Infection-associated
        Viral infection
        Syphilis
        Tuberculosis
        Toxoplasmosis, other protozoan or fungal infections
        Trichinosis, other helminthic infections
    Associated with connective-tissue disease (e.g., systemic
           lupus erythematosus, rheumatoid arthritis,
           Sjögren's syndrome)
    Associated with carcinoma
    Idiopathic
Cervical spondylosis
Ankylosing spondylitis
Paget's disease
Pott's disease
Subacute combined degeneration of the spinal cord
Neurosyphilis (syphilitic meningomyelitis, tabes dorsalis)
Spinal arachnoiditis (e.g., after subarachnoid hemorrhage,
           meningitis, subarachnoid space injection)
Chronic epidural infection or granuloma (e.g., tuberculous,
           parasitic, fungal)
Electrical or radiation injury of spinal cord
Multiple sclerosis
Syringomyelia
Amyotrophic lateral sclerosis

Childhood (or Young Adulthood) Onset
Congenital
    Cerebral spastic diplegia
    Anomalies of spinal cord or vertebrae
Hereditary disease
    Werdnig-Hoffmann disease
    Muscular dystrophies
    Friedreich's ataxia
    Chronic polyneuropathies

Niemann-Pick disease
Tay-Sachs disease

References
1. Clacy RK, Aminoff MJ: Weakness, Abnormal Movements and Imbalance, p. 107. See Bibliography, 5.
2. Sweeney VP: Approach to the Patient with Sensory Loss and Weakness, p. 2361. See Bibliography, 3.

11-O. Hemiplegia (Hemiparesis)

Cerebrovascular accident (See 11-N)
    Thrombosis
    Embolism
    Hemorrhage
    Arteriovenous malformation
Transient ischemic attack
Migraine syndrome
Head trauma (e.g., brain contusion, subdural or epidural hematoma)
Todd's paralysis
Brain tumor (primary or metastatic)
Infection (e.g., brain abscess, encephalitis, subdural empyema, meningitis)
Nonketotic hyperosmolar coma
Hypertensive encephalopathy
Vasculitis
Demyelinating disease (e.g., multiple sclerosis, acute necrotizing myelitis)
Hereditary disease (e.g., leukodystrophies)
Congenital, perinatal injury
Sarcoidosis

References
1. Rowland LP: The Syndromes Caused by Weak Muscles, p. 47. See Bibliography, 2.
2. Motor Paralysis, p. 39. See Bibliography, 1.

11-P. Peripheral Neuropathy

Primary Motor, Acute (May Have Sensory Involvement)
Guillain-Barré syndrome
Infectious mononucleosis
Viral hepatitis
Porphyria
Diphtheria
Toxins (e.g., organophosphorous compounds, thallium, and
         vaccine for rabies, typhoid, smallpox)

Sensorimotor, Subacute
Alcoholism with associated nutritional deficiency
Beriberi
Other vitamin deficiencies (B_2, B_3, B_6, B_{12}, E)
Drugs, toxins
   Arsenic
   Mercury
   Thallium
   Lithium
   Gold
   Platinum
   Acrylamide
   Lead
   Industrial solvents
   Carbon monoxide
   Neuromuscular blockers (prolonged use)
   Nitrofurantoin
   Vincristine
   Hydralazine
   Metronidazole
   Phenytoin
   Isoniazid
   Ethionamide
   Disulfiram
   Cisplatin
   Amiodarone
   Thalidomide
   Taxol
   Suramin
   Chloramphenicol
   Pyroxidine
   Dapsone
   Doxorubicin

   Colchicine
   Chloroquine
   Nucleosides (ddC, ddI)
Diabetes mellitus
Atherosclerosis
Vasculitis (e.g., polyarteritis nodosa, systemic lupus erythe-
           matosus, Wegener's granulomatosis, rheumatoid
           arthritis)
Sarcoidosis
Subacute asymmetric idiopathic polyneuritis
Nonsystemic vasculitic neuropathy

Sensorimotor, Chronic
Carcinoma, lymphoma, leukemia
Amyloidosis
Paraproteinemia (especially multiple myeloma, macroglobu-
           linemia, cryoglobulinemia)
Uremia
Beriberi
Alcoholism
Diabetes mellitus
Lyme disease
HIV infection
Ischemia
Critical illness neuropathy
Connective-tissue disease (especially systemic lupus
           erythematosus)
Myxedema
Leprosy
Chronic inflammatory demyelinating polyradiculoneuropathy
Hereditary disease
   Charcot-Marie-Tooth disease
   Hereditary sensory and autonomic neuropathies
   Dejerine-Sottas disease
   Hereditary neuropathy with lability to pressure palsies
   Refsum's disease
   Abetalipoproteinemia and Tangier disease
   Metachromatic leukodystrophy
   Roussy-Lévy syndrome
   Fabry's disease
   Familial dysautonomia (Riley-Day syndrome)
   Familial amyloid neuropathies
   Ataxia telangiectasia
   Porphyric neuropathies

References
1. Adams, p. 1117. See Bibliography, 1.
2. Feosby TE: Disorders of the Peripheral Nervous System, p. 2441. See Bibliography, 3.

11-Q. Carpal Tunnel Syndrome

Idiopathic
Fibrosis or tenosynovitis of flexor tendons
Fracture (e.g., Colles')
Occupational trauma (e.g., jackhammer or keyboard operation)
Degenerative arthritis
Wrist ganglion or benign tumor
Pregnancy
Congestive heart failure (with edema)
Amyloidosis (e.g., multiple myeloma)
Rheumatoid arthritis
Scleroderma
Systemic lupus erythematosus
Diabetes mellitus
Hypothyroidism
Tuberculosis, other granulomatous diseases (e.g., leprosy, sarcoidosis)
Gout
Paget's disease
Acromegaly
Mucopolysaccharidoses
Eosinophilic fasciitis

References
1. Diseases of the Peripheral Nerves, p. 1160. See Bibliography, 1.
2. Eisen AA: Mononeuropathies Caused by Entrapment, Compression, and Other Physical Injuries, p. 2451. See Bibliography, 3.

11-R. Typical Cerebrospinal Fluid Characteristics in Various Diseases

Condition	Pressure (cm H$_2$O)	WBCs/mm^3	Predominant type of WBCs	Glucose (mg/dL)	Protein (mg/dL)	Other
Normal	5–20	<5	100% lympho-cytes	50–75% of serum value	<50	Lactate 10–20 mg/dL
Meningitis						
Bacterial	Usually ↑	100–200,000	85–95% neutro-phils	<40, or <40% of blood glucose	45–500	Lactate >35 mg/dL; positive bacterial cultures; Gram's stain, counterimmunoelectrophoresis, enzyme-linked immunosorbent assay, polymerase chain reaction
Viral	Normal to ↑	10–500	Lymphocytes (sometimes neutrophils early)	Normal, occasionally ↓	50–200	Viral cultures
Tuberculosis	↑	50–500	Lymphocytes (occasionally neutrophils)	<40	100–200	Positive mycobacterial culture or Ziehl-Neelsen stain, or both

Disease	Pressure	Cell count	Cell type	Glucose	Protein	Comments
Fungal (± abscess)	Normal to ↑	25–1,000	Lymphocytes	20–40	25–500	Antibody, antigen, and fungal preps are often useful
Neurosyphilis (meningo-vascular or paretic)	Normal to ↑	200–500	Lymphocytes	Normal	40–200	↑γ-Globulins, positive serologic tests (VDRL test usually, fluorescent treponemal antibody absorption test)
Herpes encephalitis	Normal to ↑	20–500	Lymphocytes	Normal, sometimes ↓	50–100	↑ RBCs, xanthochromia polymerase chain reaction for herpes, DNA sometimes positive
Brain abscess[a]	↑ to ↑↑	20–300 (may be >50,000 if ruptured)	10–80% neutrophils	Normal	75–100	Lumbar puncture usually contraindicated
Neoplasm[a]	Usually ↑	<100	Lymphocytes	40–80	50–1,000	Positive cytology
Cerebral hemorrhage	Usually ↑	↑ In proportion to RBCs (may be 2,000–3,000)	Lymphocytes	Normal, occasionally ↓	↑↑ (<1,000)	↑↑ RBCs xanthochromia or gross blood
Multiple sclerosis	Normal	<100 (usually <20)	Lymphocytes	Normal	<100	↑γ-Globulins (>12% of total protein); ↑ myelin basic protein, oligo-clonal bands may be present

Continued

11-R. Typical Cerebrospinal Fluid Characteristics in Various Diseases (continued)

Condition	Pressure (cm H$_2$O)	WBCs/mm^3	Predominant type of WBCs	Glucose (mg/dL)	Protein (mg/dL)	Other
Guillain-Barré syndrome	Normal	Normal (sometimes 10–100 lymphocytes)	Lymphocytes	<80	50–1,000	Protein may be normal in first few days

$\downarrow$, decreased; $\uparrow$, increased; $\uparrow\uparrow$, greatly increased; RBCs, red blood cells.
^{a}If this diagnosis is suspected, lumbar puncture is contraindicated, at least until after computed tomography has been performed.

Reference

1. Duman S, Ginsberg SH: Spinal Fluid Findings in Disease, p. 421. See Bibliography, 4.

11-S. Dermatome Chart

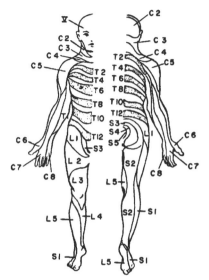

Source: Gatz AJ: *Manter's Essentials of Clinical Neuroanatomy and Neurophysiology*, 4/e. Philadelphia: FA Davis Co, 1970, p. 23.

Bibliography

1. Adams RD, Victor M: *Principles of Neurology*, 5/e. New York: McGraw-Hill, 1993.
2. Rowland LP (ed): *Merritt's Textbook of Neurology*, 9/e. Baltimore: Williams & Wilkins, 1995.
3. Kelley WN: *Textbook of Internal Medicine*, 3/e. Philadelphia: Lippincott–Raven, 1997.
4. Friedman HH: *Problem-Oriented Medical Diagnosis*, 6/e. Philadelphia: Little, Brown and Company, 1996.
5. Wilson JD, et al. (eds): *Harrison's Principles of Internal Medicine*, 14/e. New York: McGraw-Hill, 1998.
6. Plum F, Posner JB: *Dignosis of Stupor and Coma*, 3/e. Philadelphia: FA Davis Co, 1980.

12 RESPIRATORY SYSTEM

12-A. Cough

Acute
Viral upper respiratory infection
  Pharyngitis
  Rhinitis
  Tracheobronchitis
  Bronchiolitis
  Serous otitis
Gastroesophageal reflux
Bacterial and other infections
  Tracheobronchitis
  Bordetella pertussis
  Sinusitis, especially maxillary
  Otitis media or externa
  Pneumonia
  Lung abscess
Asthma
Inhalation of irritants (environmental, occupational)
  Smoke/smog
  Noxious fumes
  Extremely hot or cold air
Pulmonary edema
Pulmonary embolism
Aspiration pneumonitis
Foreign body inhalation
Laryngeal inflammation
External or middle ear disease

Acute pleural, pericardial, mediastinal, or diaphragmatic
        inflammation

Chronic
(May have more than one etiology)
Postnasal drip syndrome
    Chronic bacterial sinusitis
    Perennial nonallergic rhinitis
    Perennial or seasonal allergic rhinitis
    Vasomotor rhinitis
    Postinfectious rhinitis
    Allergic fungal sinusitis
    Nonallergic rhinitis
        Medication abuse (legal or illegal)
        Environmental irritants
        Pregnancy
Asthma
Gastroesophageal reflux
Bronchiectasis
Neoplasms (especially endobronchial or laryngeal), malig-
        nant and benign
Lung abscess
Interstitial lung disease (see 12-N)
Recurrent aspiration
    Hiatal hernia
    Achalasia
Drug-induced
    Angiotensin-converting enzyme inhibitors
    Beta blockers, selective and nonselective
    Amiodarone
Chronic pulmonary edema
Mitral stenosis
Chronic laryngeal inflammation or tumor
Chronic pneumonia, especially tuberculous and fungal
Cystic fibrosis
External and middle-ear disease, chronic
Miscellaneous
    Bronchogenic/mediastinal cyst
    Zenker's diverticulum
    Aortic aneurysm
    Irritation of vagal afferent nerve
    Osteophytes
    Pacemaker wires
    Chronic pleural, pericardial, mediastinal, or diaphragmatic
            inflammation
Psychogenic/habit cough

References

1. See Bibliography, 4.
2. Braman SS, Corrao WM: Cough: Differential Diagnosis and Treatment. *Clin Chest Med* 8:177, 1987.
3. Thompson BT, Kazemi H: Pulmonary Problems, p. 168. See Bibliography, 1.

12-B. Dyspnea

Acute
Pleuropulmonary causes
    Obstructive lung disease
    Asthma
    Acute tracheobronchitis
    Pneumonitis
    Pulmonary edema and congestion (see 12-L)
    Pulmonary thromboembolism/vasculitis
    Pneumothorax
    Pleurisy and/or pleural effusion
    Gastric or other fluid aspiration
    Noxious gas inhalation (including carbon monoxide)
    Upper airway obstruction (see 12-C)
    Collapse of lung segment(s)
    Angioedema
    Foreign-body aspiration
    Chest trauma
        Pulmonary contusion
        Rib fractures
        Flail chest
Nonpulmonary causes
    Psychogenic disorders (e.g., anxiety)
    Decreased inspired oxygen tension (e.g., at high altitude)
    Acute neuromuscular dysfunction
    Shock
    Fever
    Acute anemia
    Increased intracranial pressure
    Metabolic acidosis
    Cardiac tamponade

Chronic
Pleuropulmonary causes
    Chronic obstructive pulmonary disease

      Chronic bronchitis
      Emphysema
      Cystic fibrosis
   Asthma
   Pulmonary edema or congestion (see 12-L)
   Interstitial fibrosis (any cause)
   Chronic pneumonia
   Pulmonary vascular disease
      Recurrent pulmonary emboli
      Pulmonary hypertension
      Arteriovenous malformation
   Malignancy
      Bronchogenic carcinoma
      Pulmonary metastatic disease
   Respiratory muscle disease
      Phrenic nerve dysfunction
      Neuromuscular disease
         Myasthenia gravis
         Poliomyelitis
         Guillain-Barré syndrome
         Muscular dystrophy
   Chest wall abnormalities
      Pectus excavatum
      Kyphoscoliosis
   Pleural disease
      Effusion
      Fibrothorax
      Primary or metastatic neoplasm
   Bronchiectasis
   Alveolar filling disease
      Pulmonary alveolar proteinosis
      Alveolar microlithiasis
      Lipoid pneumonia
   Lung resection
   Upper airway obstruction
Nonpulmonary causes
   Anemia
   Obesity
   Psychogenic disorders
   Abdominal mass (e.g. tumor, pregnancy)
   Ascites
   Metabolic acidosis
   Thyroid disease
   Arteriovenous shunt
   Congenital heart disease
   Abnormal hemoglobin

References
1. Ingram RH, Braunwald E: Dyspnea and Pulmonary Edema, pp. 190–194. See Bibliography, 3.
2. Stulbarg MS, Adams L: Dyspnea, pp. 511–528. See Bibliography, 5.
3. See Bibliography, 6.

12-C. Wheezing

Asthma
Extrinsic
Intrinsic
Exercise- or cold-induced
Drug-induced
    Aspirin
    Beta blockers
    Acetylcysteine
    Indomethacin
    Tartrazine

Other Etiologies
Peripheral airway obstruction
    Bronchitis, chronic or acute
    Bronchiolitis
    Bronchiectasis
    Cystic fibrosis
    Pneumonia
Pulmonary embolism
Cardiac asthma (see 12-L)
Aspiration
    Foreign body
    Gastric contents
Irritant inhalants
    Toluene diisocyanate
    Sulfur dioxide
Anaphylaxis
Upper airway obstruction
    Extrinsic
        Thyroid enlargement, tumor, hemorrhage
        Lymphoma
        Edema of, or hemorrhage into, subcutaneous tissues
            of neck
        Retropharyngeal edema, hemorrhage, abscess

    Intrinsic
        Epiglottitis
        Foreign body
        Tracheal fracture, stricture, tracheomalacia
        Laryngeal tumor, trauma, edema, spasm
        Vocal cord dysfunction or paralysis
        Amyloidosis
    Functional
        Laryngeal dyskinesia
Large airway obstruction
    Extrinsic
        Mediastinal hemorrhage or tumor
        Esophageal cancer
        Vascular compression
            Aortic aneurysm
            Congenital anomalies
    Intrinsic
        Tracheal stricture, tumor, tracheomalacia
Pulmonary infiltrates with eosinophilia
    Loeffler's syndrome
    Tropical eosinophilia
    Chronic eosinophilic pneumonia
    Bronchopulmonary aspergillosis
    Polyarteritis nodosa
Angioedema
    Idiopathic
    Hereditary angioneurotic edema
Carcinoid syndrome

References

1. Thompson BT, Kazemi H: Pulmonary Problems, p. 173. See Bibliography, 1.
2. Hollingsworth HM: Wheezing and Stridor. *Clin Chest Med* 8:231–240, 1987.

12-D. Hemoptysis*

Pseudohemoptysis
Blood of upper gastrointestinal origin
Upper airway lesions
    Epistaxis
    Gingival bleeding
    Oropharyngeal carcinoma

Laryngeal carcinoma or other lesions
Hereditary hemorrhagic telangiectasia
Serratia marcescens infection
Airway trauma

Tracheobronchial Sources
Bronchitis, chronic or acute
Bronchiectasis
Bronchogenic carcinoma
Bronchial adenoma
Foreign body
Endobronchial metastatic neoplasm
Bronchial trauma
Cystic fibrosis
Broncholithiasis
Amyloidosis

Pulmonary Parenchymal Sources
Pneumonia
    Bacterial
    Tuberculous
Pulmonary embolism/infarction
Neoplasm
Lung abscess
Fungal infections (especially aspergilloma)
Lung contusion or laceration
Goodpasture's syndrome
Wegener's granulomatosis
Idiopathic pulmonary hemosiderosis
Inhalation injury (toxic gases)
Sequestration
Bronchogenic cyst
Parasitic infestation (e.g., *Paragonimus westermani*)
Pulmonary endometriosis

Cardiac or Vascular Disorders
Pulmonary edema and congestion
Severe mitral stenosis
Aortic aneurysm
Primary pulmonary hypertension
Arteriovenous malformation
Eisenmenger's syndrome
Pulmonary vasculitis
Collagen vascular diseases (lupus)
Behçet's syndrome

Pulmonary venoocclusive disease
Pulmonary telangiectasia

Hematologic Disorders
Coagulopathy
  Congenital
  Acquired, including anticoagulant therapy
Thrombocytopenia (see 8-J)

References
1. Weinberger SE, Braunwald E: Cough and Hemoptysis, pp. 194–198. See Bibliography, 3.
2. Cahill BC, Ingbar DH: Massive Hemoptysis. *Clin Chest Med* 15:147, 1994.
3. Israel RH, Poe RH: Hemoptysis. *Clin Chest Med* 8:197–205, 1987.

*Five percent to 15% of patients remain undiagnosed despite extensive evaluation.

12-E. Cyanosis*

Central Cyanosis
Arterial desaturation
  Decreased inspired oxygen tension
  Pulmonary disease
    Alveolar hypoventilation
    Ventilation-perfusion mismatch
    Impaired oxygen diffusion
  Anatomic (right-to-left) shunt
    Congenital heart disease
    Pulmonary arteriovenous fistulas
    Other intrapulmonary shunts
Hemoglobin abnormalities
  Methemoglobinemia
  Sulfhemoglobinemia
  Hemoglobin with low affinity for oxygen (e.g., hemoglobin Kansas)
Pseudocyanosis
  Polycythemia vera
  Argyria
  Hemochromatosis

Peripheral Cyanosis
Reduced cardiac output
Cold exposure (including Raynaud's phenomenon)
Arterial obstruction
Venous stasis and/or obstruction

References
1. Braunwald E: Cyanosis, Hypoxia, and Polycythemia, pp. 205–210. See Bibliography, 3.
2. Guenter CA: Respiratory Function of the Lungs and Blood, 179–180. See Bibliography, 7.

*Indicates ≥5 gm of unsaturated hemoglobin or ≥1.5 gm of methemoglobin present.

12-F. Pleuritic Pain*

Chest Wall Disease
Bony thorax
    Costochondritis (Tietze's syndrome)
    Rib fracture or tumor
    Fractured cartilage
    Periostitis
    Periosteal hematoma
    Xiphoidalgia
    Thoracic spondylitis due to arthritis, infection, trauma
Soft tissues
    Infection
    Muscle spasm (intercostal or pectoral)
    Myositis
    Fibromyositis
Neural structures
    Intercostal neuritis
    Herpes zoster
    Neurofibromatosis
    Causalgia
    Anterior chest wall syndrome

Pleuropulmonary Disease[†]
Infectious pleuritis, especially viral
Idiopathic pleurodynia
Pulmonary embolism and infarction

Pneumonia
Pneumothorax
Trauma
Neoplasm
    Primary
    Metastatic
    Direct invasion
Immune-mediated disease
    Systemic lupus erythematosus
    Postcardiac injury syndrome
    Rheumatoid arthritis
    Vasculitis
Diaphragmatic irritation
    Pancreatitis
    Abscess (subphrenic, splenic, hepatic)
Asbestosis
Uremic pleuritis
Radiation pleuritis
Familial polyserositis
Middle lobe syndrome

Mediastinal Disease
Pneumomediastinum
Mediastinitis
Esophageal perforation
Esophageal variceal sclerotherapy
Pericarditis
Tumor, primary or metastatic

References
1. See Bibliography, 8.
2. Thompson BT, Kazemi H: Pulmonary Problems, pp. 171–173. See Bibliography, 1.
3. Donat WE: Chest Pain: Cardiac and Noncardiac Causes. *Clin Chest Med* 8:241–252, 1987.

*Pleuritic pain is defined as pain accentuated by breathing, coughing, or sneezing.
†Most of the disorders that cause exudative effusions also cause pleuritic pain. See 12-G for a more complete list.

12-G. Pleural Effusion: Exudate

Exudative Pleural Effusion
Infection
  Bacterial
    Empyema (see 12-J)
    Parapneumonic effusion
  Tuberculous
  Viral
  Fungal
  Parasitic (amebiasis, echinococcosis, paragonimiasis)
  Mycoplasma, actinomycosis, nocardiosis
  Rickettsiae (Q fever)
Neoplasm
  Lung*
  Breast*
  Lymphoma*
  Ovarian neoplasm (Meigs' syndrome)
  Metastases (sarcoma, melanoma)
  Kaposi's sarcoma
  Primary pleural malignancy
Thromboembolic disease
  Pulmonary embolism
  Pulmonary infarction
Immune-mediated diseases
  Rheumatoid disease
  Systemic lupus erythematosus
  Churg-Strauss syndrome
  Drug-induced lupus
  Wegener's granulomatosis
  Sarcoidosis
  Postcardiac injury syndrome
  Angioimmunoblastic lymphadenopathy
  Sjögren's syndrome
  Eosinophilia-myalgia syndrome
  Familial Mediterranean fever
Intraabdominal disorders
  Pancreatitis
  Esophageal perforation
  Intraabdominal abscesses (e.g., hepatic, splenic,
        subphrenic)
  After liver transplants
  Esophageal variceal sclerotherapy
  Post–abdominal surgery
  Postpartum state

Drug-induced pleural disease
  Nitrofurantoin
  Methysergide
  Dantrolene
  Bromocriptine
  Interleukin 2
  Procarbazine
  Methotrexate
  Amiodarone
Inhalation of inorganic dusts
  Asbestosis
Other causes
  Yellow nail syndrome
  Uremic pleuritis
  Radiation pleuritis
  Myxedema
  Spontaneous pneumothorax
  Trapped lung
  Postpartum pleural effusion
  Amyloidosis
  Ovarian hyperstimulation

Hemothorax
Traumatic
  Penetrating or nonpenetrating trauma
  Iatrogenic
Nontraumatic
  Malignancy, especially metastatic
  Anticoagulant therapy for pulmonary emboli
  Spontaneous
    Secondary to bleeding disorder (hemophilia, thrombo-
        cytopenia)
    Rupture of intrathoracic vessel or aneurysm
    Ruptured pancreatic pseudocyst
    Thoracic endometriosis
    Idiopathic
  Pulmonary emboli

Chylothorax
Traumatic
  Penetrating or nonpenetrating trauma
  Surgery
  Iatrogenic
Malignancy (causes 50% of chylothoraces)
  Lymphoma (accounts for 75% of malignant chylothoraces)
  Metastatic malignancy

Kaposi's sarcoma in acquired immunodeficiency
syndrome (AIDS)
Thrombosis of superior vena cava/subclavian vein
Idiopathic
Congenital
Pulmonary lymphangiomyomatosis
Pseudochylothorax

References

1. Connors AF, Altose MD: Pleural Disease, p. 1839. See
   Bibliography, 9.
2. See Bibliography, 10.

*Causes 75% of malignant pleural effusions.

12-H. Pleural Effusion: Transudate

Cardiac disease
   Congestive heart failure
   Fluid overload
   Constrictive pericarditis
   Obstruction of superior vena cava or azygos vein
Renal disease
   Nephrotic syndrome
   Acute glomerulonephritis
   Urinary tract obstruction
   Peritoneal dialysis
Liver disease
   Cirrhosis with ascites
Thromboembolic disease
   Pulmonary embolism*
Others
   Meigs' syndrome*
   Myxedema*
   Sarcoidosis
   Severe malnutrition (with hypoalbuminemia)
   Iatrogenic (e.g., venous catheter in pleural space)
   After lung transplantation

References

1. Connors AF, Altose MD: Pleural Disease, p. 1839. See
   Bibliography, 9.
2. Light, pp. 83–93. See Bibliography, 10.

*Most are exudates.

12-I. Pleural Effusion: Exudate versus Transudate*

Characteristics of an exudative effusion
    Pleural fluid–serum protein ratio >0.5
    Pleural fluid lactic dehydrogenase (LDH) greater than two-
        thirds of the upper limit of normal for serum LDH
    Pleural fluid–serum LDH ratio >0.6

References
1. Light RW, et al: Pleural Effusions: The Diagnostic
   Separation of Transudates and Exudates. *Ann Intern Med*
   77:507, 1972.
2. See Bibliography, 10.

*An exudate has one or more of these three characteristics; a transu-
date does not have any of these characteristics.

12-J. Empyema

Pulmonary Causes
Pneumonia (anaerobic more than aerobic bacteria)
Bronchial obstruction
    Tumor
    Foreign body
Hematogenous spread of infection
Bronchopleural fistula
Ruptured abscess
Spontaneous pneumothorax
Bronchiectasis
Rheumatoid disease

Mediastinal Causes
Esophageal perforation
Abscess
    Lymph node
    Osteomyelitis
    Pericarditis

Subdiaphragmatic Causes
Abscess (hepatic, pancreatic, splenic, retrogastric)
Peritonitis

Direct Inoculation
Postoperative
    Infected hemothorax
    Leaky bronchial stump (postlobectomy or postpneu-
          monectomy)
Penetrating chest trauma
    Foreign body in pleural space
Iatrogenic inoculation
    Thoracentesis
    Chest tube

References

1. Snider GL, Saleh SS: Empyema of the Thorax in Adults:
   Review of 105 Cases. *Chest* 54:410, 1968.
2. See Bibliography, 10.

12-K. Pneumothorax

Primary spontaneous pneumothorax
Secondary spontaneous pneumothorax
    Obstructive pulmonary disease
        Chronic airway obstruction
        Asthma
    Malignancy
        Primary lung carcinoma
        Pleural metastatic disease
    Infectious disease
        Lung abscess
        Tuberculosis
        Pneumocystis carinii in patients with AIDS
    Pulmonary infarction
    Diffuse lung disease
        Idiopathic pulmonary fibrosis
        Eosinophilic granuloma
        Scleroderma
        Rheumatoid disease
        Tuberous sclerosis
        Sarcoidosis
        Lymphangiomyomatosis
        Idiopathic pulmonary hemosiderosis
        Alveolar proteinosis
        Xanthomatosis
        Biliary cirrhosis

    Pneumoconiosis
        Silicosis
        Berylliosis
    Congenital disease
        Cystic fibrosis
        Marfan's syndrome
    Catamenial pneumothorax
    Neonatal pneumothorax
Iatrogenic pneumothorax
Traumatic pneumothorax
    Penetrating thoracic trauma
    Barotrauma
    Sudden chest compression
    Blunt abdominal trauma
    Drug abuse (attempted injection in subclavian/internal
        jugular vein)

Reference
1. See Bibliography, 10.

12-L. Pulmonary Edema

Elevated Microvascular Pressure
Cardiogenic (see 2-G)
Volume overload (especially when associated with low
        plasma oncotic pressure)
Neurogenic
    Head trauma
    Intracerebral hemorrhage
    Postictal
Pulmonary venous obstruction
    Chronic mediastinitis
    Anomalous pulmonary venous return
    Congenital pulmonary venous stenosis
    Idiopathic venoocclusive disease

Normal Microvascular Pressure
(Adult Respiratory Distress Syndrome)
Infection
    Sepsis
    Pneumonia
        Bacterial

    Viral
    Mycoplasmal
    Fungal
    P. carinii
    Legionnaires' disease
  Miliary tuberculosis
  Toxic shock syndrome
  Malaria
Liquid aspiration
  Gastric contents
  Water (near-drowning, fresh and saltwater)
  Hypertonic contrast media
  Ethyl alcohol
Shock, especially septic (see 2-K)
Multiple trauma and burns
Hematologic disorders
  Diffuse intravascular coagulation
  Transfusion-related leukoagglutinins
  Leukemia
  Thrombotic thrombocytopenic purpura
  Unfiltered blood transfusion (controversial)
Inhaled toxic gases
  Oxygen (high concentration)
  Smoke
  Nitrogen dioxide
  Sulfur dioxide
  Chlorine
  Phosgene
  Ozone
  Metallic oxides
  Acid fumes
  Carbon monoxide
  Hydrocarbons
  Cadmium
  Ammonia
Embolism
  Thrombus
  Fat
  Air
  Amniotic fluid
Acute pancreatitis
Drug overdose
  Narcotics
  Propoxyphene
  Chlordiazepoxide
  Aspirin

Ethchlorvynol
Barbiturates
Colchicine
Drug-induced lung injury (see 12-N)
Paraquat
Nitrofurantoin
Amiodarone
Immunologic injury
Goodpasture's syndrome
Systemic lupus erythematosus
Associated with high negative pleural pressure
Postthoracentesis
Post–expansion of pneumothorax
Acute bronchial asthma
Complete upper airway obstruction (e.g., hanging)
Pulmonary lymphatic obstruction
Fibrotic and inflammatory disease (e.g., silicosis)
Lymphangitic carcinomatosis
Post–lung transplant
Miscellaneous
Acute radiation pneumonitis
Pulmonary contusion
Post–cardiopulmonary bypass
Diabetic ketoacidosis
Circulating vasoactive substance (e.g., histamine)
Dextran
Lymphangiogram dye (mechanism controversial)
Eclampsia

Unclear Mechanisms
High-altitude pulmonary edema

References
1. Honig EG, Ingram RH: Acute Respiratory Distress Syndrome, p. 1483. See Bibliography, 3.
2. Matthay MA, Hopewell PC: Critical Care for Acute Respiratory Failure. See Bibliography, 9.
3. Hudson LD: Causes of the Adult Respiratory Distress Syndrome: Clinical Recognition. *Clin Chest Med* 3:195, 1982.

12-M. Respiratory Failure

Central Nervous System Disorders
Drug intoxication
  Sedatives
  Tranquilizers
  Analgesics
  Anesthetics
Vascular disorders, hypoperfusion states
  Intracranial infarction or bleeding (especially brainstem)
  Shock (see 2-K)
Disorders of the central respiratory controller
  Primary alveolar hypoventilation
  Obstructive sleep apnea syndrome
Trauma
  Spinal cord injury
  Head injury
  Increased intracranial pressure
Infection
  Viral encephalitis
  Bulbar poliomyelitis
Miscellaneous
  Status epilepticus
  Myxedema

Neuromuscular Disorders
Peripheral nerve and anterior horn cell disorders
  Guillain-Barré syndrome
  Poliomyelitis
  Amyotrophic lateral sclerosis
Myoneural junction disorders
  Myasthenia gravis
  Tetanus
  Curarelike drugs
  Anticholinesterase drugs
Muscular disorders
  Muscle weakness due to, for example, hypophos-
        phatemia, hypokalemia
  Muscle fatigue
  Polymyositis, dermatomyositis
  Muscular dystrophies
  Myotonia

Chest Wall and Pleural Disorders
Kyphoscoliosis
Chest trauma
    Flail chest
    Multiple rib fractures
    Postthoracotomy
Pleural disorders
    Large pleural effusions (see 12-G, 12-H)
    Tension pneumothorax
    Massive fibrosis

Pulmonary Disorders
Airflow limitation, chronic
    Pulmonary emphysema
    Chronic bronchitis
    Asthma, especially status asthmaticus
Alveolar disorders
    Pneumonia
    Aspiration pneumonitis
    Pulmonary edema (see 12-L)
        Elevated microvascular pressure
        Normal microvascular pressure (adult respiratory distress syndrome)
    Combined or unclear mechanisms
Airway obstruction, acute
    Foreign body
    Upper airway obstruction (see 12-C)
    Epiglottitis
    Respiratory burns
    Noxious gases
    Bronchospasm, acute (see 12-C)
Interstitial disorders
    Fibrosing alveolitis
    Interstitial fibrosis and other diffuse disorders (see 12-N)
    Extensive neoplasm
Vascular disorders
    Pulmonary embolus (especially thrombus, fat)
    Obliterative vasculitis
        Primary pulmonary hypertension
        Scleroderma

References
1. Matthay MA, Hopewell PC: Critical Care for Acute Respiratory Failure, pp. 379–396. See Bibliography, 9.
2. Pontoppidan H, Geffin B, Lowenstein E: Acute Respiratory Failure. N Engl J Med 287:690, 743, 799, 1972.

12-N. Interstitial Lung Disease

Interstitial Disease of Known Etiology

Inorganic dusts
  Silica
  Silicates, especially asbestos, talc, kaolin,
        diatomaceous earth
  Aluminum
    Powdered aluminum
    Bauxite
  Antimony
  Carbon
    Coal
    Granite
  Beryllium
  Mixed dusts
  Metal dusts, especially titanium, tungsten, cadmium
Organic dusts (hypersensitivity pneumonitis)
  Farmer's lung
  Humidifier lung
  Bagassosis
  Many others (see reference 2)
Gases, fumes, vapors, aerosols
  Gases
    Oxygen
    Sulfur dioxide
    Chlorine gas
  Fumes
    Oxides of zinc, cadmium, copper, and others
    Mercury
    Toluene diisocyanate
  Aerosols
    Fats
    Pyrethrum
    Bordeaux mixture
Drugs
  Chemotherapeutic agents
    Busulfan
    Bleomycin
    Cyclophosphamide
    Methotrexate
    Nitrosoureas
    Procarbazine
    Mitomycin
  Antibiotics
    Nitrofurantoin

      Sulfonamides
      Penicillin
   Others
      Diphenylhydantoin
      Drugs causing drug-induced lupus
      Gold salts
      Amiodarone
      Methysergide
      Carbamazepine
      Propranolol
Poisons
   Paraquat
Infections
Radiation injury (acute or chronic)
Graft-versus-host reaction
Chronic pulmonary edema
Chronic uremia
Adult respiratory distress syndrome (see 12-L)

Interstitial Disease of Unknown Etiology
Idiopathic pulmonary fibrosis
Sarcoidosis
Collagen vascular disease/autoimmune diseases
   Rheumatoid arthritis
   Progressive systemic sclerosis
   Systemic lupus erythematosus
   Polymyositis-dermatomyositis
   Sjögren's syndrome
Vasculitis
   Wegener's granulomatosis
   Lymphomatoid granulomatosis
   Churg-Strauss syndrome
   Hypersensitivity vasculitis
   Overlap syndromes
Eosinophilic lung disease
   Eosinophilic granuloma
   Chronic eosinophilic pneumonia
   Hypereosinophilic syndrome
Idiopathic pulmonary hemosiderosis
Goodpasture's syndrome
Immunoblastic lymphadenopathy
Lymphocytic interstitial pneumonitis
Lymphangiomyomatosis
Amyloidosis
Alveolar proteinosis
Bronchocentric granulomatosis

Inherited disorders
    Familial interstitial fibrosis
    Tuberous sclerosis
    Neurofibromatosis
    Hermansky-Pudlak syndrome
    Niemann-Pick disease
    Gaucher's disease
Liver disease
    Chronic active hepatitis
    Primary biliary cirrhosis
Bowel disease
    Whipple's disease
    Ulcerative colitis
    Crohn's disease
    Weber-Christian disease

References

1. Reynolds HY: Interstitial Lung Diseases, p. 1095. See Bibliography, 3.
2. Fulmer JD, Katzenstein AA: The Interstitial Lung Diseases, pp. 1–15, section L. See Bibliography, 11.
3. King TE, Chemisck RM, Schwarz MI: IP F and other Interstitial Lung Diseases of Unknown Etiology, pp. 1827–1849. See Bibliography, 5.

12-O. Pulmonary Hypertension

Pulmonary Arterial Hypertension (Precapillary)

Alveolar hypoxemia with vasoconstriction
    Most causes of respiratory failure (see 12-M)
    Chronic obstructive lung disease
        Chronic bronchitis/bronchiolitis
        Emphysema
        Asthma
        Cystic fibrosis
        Bronchiectasis
    Alveolar disorders
        Pneumonia
        Aspiration pneumonitis
        Pulmonary edema (see 12-L)
        Chronic alveolar filling disorders
    Upper airway obstruction (see 12-C)
    Alveolar hypoventilation

    Neuromuscular disorders (see 11-D)
    Central nervous system disorders (see 12-M)
    Obesity
    Primary alveolar hypoventilation
    Obstructive sleep apnea syndrome
  Chest wall and pleural disorders
    Chest deformity
      Kyphoscoliosis
      Thoracoplasty
      Poliomyelitis
      Muscular dystrophy
    Pleural disease (especially fibrothorax)
  High-altitude pulmonary hypertension
Restriction of the vascular bed
  Extrinsic
    Diffuse interstitial disease (see 12-N)
      Sarcoidosis
      Other granulomatous diseases
      Interstitial fibrosis
    Neoplasm
      Metastatic
      Alveolar cell carcinoma
  Intrinsic
    Pulmonary thromboembolic disease
      Thrombotic
      Metastatic neoplasm
      Septic
      Fat
      Foreign material (e.g., talc)
      Amniotic fluid
      Antiphospholipid syndrome
      Parasitic
        Schistosomiasis
        Filariasis
    Pulmonary arteritis
      Raynaud's syndrome
      Scleroderma
      Calcinosis cutis, Raynaud's phenomenon,
        esophageal dysfunction, sclerodactyly, and
        telangiectasia (CREST) syndrome
      Rheumatoid disease
      Systemic lupus erythematosus
      Polymyositis, dermatomyositis
      Takayasu's arteritis
      Granulomatous arteritis
    Toxin-induced pulmonary vascular

        Intravenous drug use
        Cocaine use
        L-Tryptophan
        Anorexic agents
     Thrombosis due to sickle cell disease
     Human immunodeficiency virus–associated pulmonary
        hypertension
  Increased flow
     Patent ductus arteriosus
     Atrial septal defect
        Eisenmenger's physiology
     Ventricular septal defect
     Sinus of Valsalva aneurysm
  Decreased flow
     Tetralogy of Fallot
Destruction of vascular bed (e.g., emphysema)
Primary pulmonary hypertension

Pulmonary Venous Hypertension (Postcapillary)

Cardiac disease
  Left ventricular failure (see 2-G)
  Mitral valve disease
     Mitral stenosis
     Mitral insufficiency
  Left atrial obstruction
     Myxoma or other tumor
     Supravalvular stenotic ring
     Thrombus
  Cor triatriatum
Pericardial disease
  Pericardial tamponade
  Restrictive pericarditis
Pulmonary venous disease
  Mediastinal neoplasm or granuloma
  Mediastinal fibrosis
  Mediastinitis
  Anomalous pulmonary venous return
  Congenital pulmonary venous stenosis
  Idiopathic pulmonary venoocclusive disease

References

1. Fraser, p. 1833. See Bibliography, 2.
2. Greenberg HE, Scharf SM. Pulmonary Hypertension: Pathophysiology and Clinical Disorders, pp. 1285–1304. See Bibliography, 9.

3. Rich S: Primary Pulmonary Hypertension, pp. 1466–1468. See Bibliography, 3.
4. Mitzner WA: Pulmonary Circulation: General Principles and Dx Approach, L-2, p. 2. See Bibliography, 11.

12-P. Mediastinal Masses by Predominant Compartment

Anterior
Substernal thyroid
Thymoma
Lymphoma
Germinal cell neoplasm (e.g., dermoid)
Ascending aortic aneurysm
Parathyroid tumor
Mesenchymal neoplasm (e.g., lipoma or fibroma)
Hematoma
Bronchogenic cyst

Middle
Lymphoma
Metastatic neoplasm (pulmonary or extrapulmonary)
Sarcoid lymphadenopathy
Infectious granulomatous disease
Bronchogenic cyst
Vascular dilatation
    Superior vena cava
    Azygos vein
    Pulmonary artery
Aortic arch aneurysm
Vascular anomaly
Pleuropericardial cyst
Lymph node hyperplasia
Mononucleosis-associated adenopathy
Primary or tracheal neoplasm
Hematoma

Anterior Cardiophrenic Angle
Pleuropericardial cyst or tumor
Foramen of Morgagni hernia
Fat pad
Diaphragmatic lymph node enlargement (e.g., lymphoma)

Pulmonary parenchymal mass
Cardiac aneurysm
Pericardial fat necrosis

Posterior
Neurogenic tumor
Meningocele
Esophageal lesion
   Neoplasm
   Diverticulum
   Megaesophagus of any etiology (e.g., achalasia)
   Hiatal hernia
Bochdalek hernia
Thoracic spine lesion
   Neoplasm
   Infectious spondylitis
   Fracture with hematoma
Extramedullary hematopoiesis
Descending aortic aneurysm
Mediastinal abscess
Pancreatic pseudocyst
Lymph node hyperplasia
Hematoma
Cystic lesion
   Neurenteric cyst
   Gastroenteric cyst
   Thoracic duct
   Bronchogenic cyst

Diffuse Mediastinal Widening
Bronchogenic carcinoma
Mediastinal hemorrhage
Granulomatous mediastinitis
   Idiopathic
   Tuberculosis
   Histoplasmosis
Mediastinal lipomatosis
Pneumomediastinum
Acute mediastinitis

Reference
1. Wychulis AR, et al: Surgical Treatment of Mediastinal Tumors: A 40 Year Experience. *J Thorac Cardiovasc Surg* 62:379, 1971.

12-Q. Solitary Pulmonary Nodule

Neoplasm
    Bronchogenic carcinoma
    Metastatic malignancy
    Hamartoma
    Bronchial adenoma
    Lymphoma
    Plasmacytoma
    Amyloidosis
    Other rare neoplasms
Infection
    Tuberculosis
    Histoplasmosis
    Aspergillosis (mucoid impaction)
    Cryptococcosis
    Dirofilaria immitis
Immune disorders
    Rheumatoid nodule
    Wegener's granulomatosis
Developmental disorders
    Bronchogenic cyst
    Arteriovenous fistula
    Sequestration
    Varicose pulmonary vein
    Bronchial atresia
Other
    Pulmonary infarction
    Lipoid pneumonia
    Hematoma

Reference
1. Fraser, p. 2170. See Bibliography, 2.

12-R. Solitary Pulmonary Nodule: Distinguishing Benign from Malignant Lesions

	Benign	Malignant
CLINICAL FINDINGS		
Age*	<40	>45
Symptoms	Absent	Present
History	Tuberculosis exposure	Smoker
	Histoplasmosis exposure	Extrathoracic
	Nonsmoker	malignancy
	Mineral oil use	Prior malignancy
X-RAY FINDINGS		
Size	<2 cm	>2 cm
Border*	Smooth, well-defined	Ill-defined, lobulated
Calcification*	Laminated, "popcorn," or multiple punctate	Rare, eccentric if present
Doubling time*	<1 or >16 mo	1–16 mo

*These factors are most important in distinguishing benign from malignant lesions.

Source: Modified from Fraser RG, Paré JAP, eds: *Diagnosis of Diseases of the Chest*, 3/e. Philadelphia: Saunders, 1989, p. 1390.

12-S. Elevated Hemidiaphragm

Pseudoelevation
Subpulmonic effusion
Diaphragmatic neoplasm

True Elevation
Intrathoracic conditions
    Lobar or segmental atelectasis
    Pneumonia
    Pulmonary infarction
    Rib fracture
    Pleurisy
Paralysis or paresis due to phrenic nerve dysfunction
    Bronchogenic carcinoma or mediastinal malignancy
    Surgical or nonsurgical trauma
    Neurologic disorders
        Myelitis

       Encephalitis
       Herpes zoster
       Poliomyelitis
       Myotonia
       Serum sickness after tetanus antitoxin
       Diphtheria
     Extrinsic pressure
       Substernal thyroid
       Aortic aneurysm
     Infection
       Tuberculosis
       Pneumonia
       Empyema or pleuritis
       Infection of the neck or cervical spine
     Radiation therapy
     Idiopathic
Intraabdominal pathology
     Subphrenic or hepatic abscess
     Pancreatitis
     Other intrahepatic mass lesion, especially malignancy
     Other intraabdominal mass
     Splenic infarct
Eventration
Traumatic rupture of the diaphragm

References

1. Riley EA: Idiopathic Diaphragmatic Paralysis. *Am J Med* 32:404, 1962.
2. Felson B, p. 421. See Bibliography, 12.

12-T. Factors Associated with an Increased Risk of Postoperative Pulmonary Complications

General Factors

     Cigarette smoking (especially more than 10 years of one pack of cigarettes per day)
     Chronic bronchitis
     Older age plus concomitant illness (not age alone)
     Alcohol abuse
     Abnormal chest x-ray
Surgical factors
     Thoracic surgery (especially with resection of functional lung)
     Upper abdominal surgery

Anesthesia time exceeding 3 to 4 hours, anesthesia type
Intraoperative pancuronium
Pulmonary function (variable predictive value)
  Forced vital capacity <70% of predicted
  Forced expiratory volume in 1 second <70%
        of predicted
  Forced expiratory volume in 1 second/forced vital
        capacity <65%
  Maximum voluntary ventilation <50% of predicted
  Diffusing capacity of carbon monoxide <50%
        of predicted
  $\dot{V}O_2$max <15 mL/min/kg
Arterial blood gases
  $Paco_2$ >45 mm Hg
  Hypoxemia not a reliable indicator
Hemoglobin level >16 g/dL
Asthma
Myasthenia gravis
Spinal cord injury
Acute respiratory infections

References

1. Smetana GW: Preoperative Pulmonary Evaluation. *N Engl J Med* 340:937–944, 1999.
2. Hansen JE, Wasserman K: Preoperative Evaluation of the Surgical Patient, pp. 379–396. See Bibliography, 9.
3. Frost E: Preanesthetic Assessment of the Patient with Respiratory Disease. *Anesth Clin North Am* 8:657–677, 1990.

Bibliography

1. Samiy AH, Douglas RG, Barondess JA (eds): *Textbook of Diagnostic Medicine*. Philadelphia: Lea & Febiger, 1987.
2. Fraser RG, et al. (eds): *Diagnosis of Diseases of the Chest*, 3/e. Philadelphia: WB Saunders, 1989.
3. Fauci AS, Braunwald E, Isselbacher KJ, et al. (eds): *Harrison's Principles of Internal Medicine*, 14/e. New York: McGraw-Hill, 1997.
4. Irwin RS, Curley FJ, Grossman RF: *Diagnosis and Treatment of Symptoms of the Respiratory Tract*. Armonk, NY: Futura, 1997.

5. Murray JF, Nadle JA: *Textbook of Respiratory Disease.* Philadelphia: WB Saunders, 1994.
6. Mahler DA: *Dyspnea.* New York: Futura, 1990.
7. Guenter CA, Welch MA (eds): *Pulmonary Medicine.* Philadelphia: Lippincott, 1982.
8. Reich NE, Fremont, RE: *Chest Pain: Systemic Differentiation and Treatment.* New York: Macmillan, 1961.
9. Wolinsky E, Baum GL (eds): *Textbook of Pulmonary Diseases,* 5/e. Boston: Little, Brown and Company, 1994.
10. Light RW: *Pleural Diseases,* 3/e. Baltimore: Williams & Wilkins, 1995.
11. Bone R (ed): *Pulmonary and Critical Care Medicine.* St. Louis: Mosby, 1998.
12. Felson B: *Chest Radiology.* Philadelphia: Saunders, 1973.

13 HUMAN IMMUNODEFICIENCY VIRUS INFECTION

13-A. Infection and Fever

Infections
Bacterial
Streptococcus pneumoniae
Salmonella spp.
Haemophilus influenzae
Staphylococcus aureus
Pseudomonas aeruginosa
Moraxella catarrhalis
Rhodococcus equi
Nocardia spp.
Legionella spp.
Syphilis
Listeria
Bartonella henselae or *Bartonella quintana*
Campylobacter spp.
Shigella spp.
Clostridium difficile
Chlamydia spp.
Borrelia burgdorferi
Viral
Human immunodeficiency virus (HIV) (especially
acute infection)
Cytomegalovirus (CMV)
Herpes simplex virus (HSV), types I and II
Epstein-Barr virus (EBV)
Varicella-zoster virus (VZV)

Hepatitis A, B, C
Human papilloma virus (HPV)
Measles virus
Papovavirus, especially JC virus
Human herpesvirus 6 (HHV-6)
Protozoa
Pneumocystis carinii
Toxoplasma gondii
Cryptosporidium parvum
Microsporidia spp., especially *Enterocytozoon bieneusi,
        Encephalitozoon* spp.
Isospora belli
Giardia lamblia
Entamoeba histolytica
Babesia microti
Cyclospora cayetanenisis
Nematode
Strongyloides stercoralis
Fungal
Cryptococcus neoformans
Candida spp.
Histoplasma capsulatum
Coccidioides immitis
Aspergillus spp.
Mucormycoses
Fusarium spp.
Blastomyces
Mycobacterium
Mycobacterium tuberculosis
Mycobacterium avium complex
Mycobacterium chelonae
Mycobacterium fortuitum
Mycobacterium kansasii
*Mycobacterium marinum, Mycobacterium scrofulaceum,
        Mycobacterium genavense, Mycobacterium gor-
        donae, Mycobacterium simiae*
Mycobacterium xenopi, Mycobacterium celatum

Malignancies
Lymphoma, especially non-Hodgkin's lymphoma (NHL), cen-
        tral nervous system (CNS) lymphoma, Hodgkin's
        disease
Kaposi's sarcoma
Squamous cell cancer (especially of skin, anus)
Solid organ tumors (see 8-A)

Metastatic cancer
Carcinomatosis
Drugs
    Trimethoprim and sulfamethoxazole (TMP/SMX)
           (Bactrim, Septra)
    Sulfonamides
    Dapsone
    Phenytoin
    Penicillins
    Amphotericin B
    Barbiturates
    Clindamycin
    Interferon
    Pentamidine
    Cephalosporins
    Carbamazepine
    Tuberculosis drugs [especially isoniazid (INH), rifampin
          and streptomycin]
    Salicylates
    Bleomycin

Other
Vaccinations
Adrenal Insufficiency

References
1. Hoeprich, pp. 635–637. See Bibliography, 1.
2. Kelley, pp. 1888–1900. See Bibliography, 2.
3. Schlossberg, pp. 283–285. See Bibliography, 3.
4. Currier, JS: Pyogenic Infections, pp. 23, 205–209. See
   Bibliography, 5.
5. Mandell, pp. 536–537. See Bibliography, 8.
6. Wormser, pp. 306–308. See Bibliography, 10.
7. Sugar, pp. 16, 66–67. See Bibliography, 14.
8. Bartlett, p. 366. See Bibliography, 17.
9. Devita, pp. 204–205, 248–249. See Bibliography, 9.

13-B. Ocular Complications

Retinitis
    CMV
    Toxoplasmosis

VZV
Fungal (especially *C. neoformans* and *H. capsulatum*)
Treponema pallidum
Idiopathic
Uveitis
  T. pallidum
  Mycobacteria spp.
  VZV
  Drugs, especially rifabutin, cidofovir
Optic neuritis
  T. pallidum
  C. neoformans
Choroiditis
  P. carinii
  Mycobacteria spp.
Other
  HIV retinopathy
  Fungal endophthalmitis (*Candida* spp.)
  Herpes zoster virus (HZV) ophthalmicus
  Fungal or bacterial corneal ulcers
  Kaposi's sarcoma (conjunctivae, lid, orbit)
  NHL (lid)
  Molluscum contagiosum (conjunctivae, lid)
  HSV keratitis
  Reiter's syndrome (conjunctivitis, arthritis, urethritis or
          cervicitis)
  VZV blepharitis, conjunctivitis, keratitis

References
1. Powderly, pp. 124–132. See Bibliography, 5.
2. Devita, pp. 233, 272, 453. See Bibliography, 9.
3. Wormser, pp. 559–581. See Bibliography, 10.
4. Jabs DA: Ophthalmologic Disease, pp. 652–665. See
   Bibliography, 15.

13-C. Hematologic Complications

Red Blood Cell Disorders
Etiologies of anemia
  HIV infection
  M. avium complex infection
  Parvovirus B19 infection
  Drugs, especially
    TMP/SMX

     Sulfonamides
     Interferon or ribavirin
     Azidothymidine (AZT)
     Ganciclovir
     Pentamidine
     Dideoxycytidine (DDC) Zalcitabine
     Lamivudine (3TC) (Epivir)
Iron-deficiency anemia
Autoimmune hemolytic anemia (AIHA)
Vitamin B_{12} deficiency
Blood loss
Bone marrow infiltration with infection (especially CMV, *M. avium* complex)
Bone marrow infiltration with malignancy (especially lymphoma)
Hypersplenism
Thrombotic thrombocytopenic purpura (TTP)

White Blood Cell Disorders

Etiologies of neutropenia or leukopenia
     HIV infection
     Drugs, especially
          DDC (Zalcitabine)
          3TC (Epivir)
          TMP/SMX
          Ganciclovir
          AZT (Retrovin)
     Bone marrow infiltration with infection (especially CMV, *M. avium* complex)
     Bone marrow infiltration with malignancy (especially lymphoma)
     Hypersplenism

Platelet Disorders

Etiologies of thrombocytopenia
     HIV infection
     CMV
     Parvovirus B19
     Fungal infections (especially *Cryptococcus* and *Histoplasma*)
     M. tuberculosis and *M. avium* complex disseminated infections
     Hepatitis B and C
     HHV-6
     Thrombotic thrombocytopenic purpura (TTP)

Drugs Causing Multiple Hematologic Abnormalities in Human Immunodeficiency Virus Infection

Zidovudine (Retrovir or AZT)
Ganciclovir
TMP/SMX
Sulfonamides
Interferon-α or ribavirin, or both
Pyrimethamine
3TC (Epivir)
Antineoplastic chemotherapy
Dapsone
Didanosine (DDI)
DDC (Zalcitabine)
Amphotericin B
Pentamidine
Fluconazole
Rifabutin
Clarithromycin

References
1. Hoeprich, pp. 635–636. See Bibliography, 1.
2. Kelley, p. 1874. See Bibliography, 2.
3. Blinder MA: Hematologic Problems, pp. 158–164. See Bibliography, 5.
4. Mandell, pp. 1225–1226. See Bibliography, 8.
5. Devita, pp. 429–433. See Bibliography, 9.
6. Wormser, pp. 542–546. See Bibliography, 10.
7. Mitsuyasu RM: Hematologic Disease, pp. 666–679. See Bibliography, 15.

13-D. Malignant Complications

Kaposi's sarcoma
Lymphoma, especially NHL, primary CNS lymphoma, Hodgkin's disease
Cervical cancer
Squamous cell cancer of the skin
Anogenital neoplasia
Squamous cell carcinoma of the anus
Basal cell cancer of the skin
Seminoma

References

1. Hoeprich, p. 638. See Bibliography, 1.
2. Kelley, pp. 1895–1897. See Bibliography, 2.
3. Von Roenn JH, Tajuddin A-K: Kaposi's sarcoma, pp. 220–222. See Bibliography, 5.
4. Kaplan L: Lymphomas, pp. 228–235. See Bibliography, 5.
5. Mandell, pp. 1240–1246. See Bibliography, 5.
6. Devita, pp. 295–317, 319–330. See Bibliography, 8.
7. Wormser, pp. 457, 459, 529–540. See Bibliography, 9.
8. Bartlett, pp. 141–142. See Bibliography, 10.

13-E. Gastrointestinal Complications

Oral or Oropharynx
Infections
    Candida spp.
    HSV
    CMV
    EBV, oral hairy leukoplakia
    Cryptococcus spp.
    Histoplasma spp.
    Bacterial infections, especially gingivitis, necrotizing ulcerative periodontal disease
    Aphthous ulcers
    Squamous cell cancer
    Kaposi's sarcoma
    Lymphoma
    VZV (trigeminal dermatome)
    Human papilloma virus
    Bacillary epithelioid angiomatosis

Esophagus
Infections
    Candida spp.
    CMV
    HSV
    Idiopathic

Colitis
Infections
    Salmonella spp.
    Shigella spp.
    M. avium complex

C. parvum
Microsporidia spp.
I. belli
CMV
Campylobacter spp.
C. difficile
Giardia lamblia
Entameba histolytica
HSV
Cyanobacteria
Strongyloides stercoralis
T. gondii

Enterocolitis
Infections
   Salmonella spp.
   Campylobacter spp.
   CMV
   Shigella spp.
   Entameba histolytica
   M. tuberculosis
   M. avium complex
   C. difficile
   Adenovirus
   Vibrio spp., especially *Vulnificus* and *Parahaemolyticus*

Hepato-Biliary Tract
Infections
   C. parvum
   CMV
   M. avium complex
   M. tuberculosis
   Chronic viral hepatitis, especially B and C
   B. henselae, B. quintana
   Kaposi's sarcoma
   Candida spp.
Drugs
   TMP/SMX
   INH
   Rifampin
   Didanosine (DDI, Videx)
   Zidovudine (AZT, Retrovir)
   Pyrazinamide
   Pentamidine

Granulomatous Hepatitis
Infections
  Mycobacteria (*M. tuberculosis, M. avium* complex)
  H. capsulatum
  C. neoformans
  Coccidioides immitis
  CMV
  P. carinii

Sclerosing Cholangitis
Infections
  C. parvum
  Microsporidia spp.
  CMV

Pancreatitis
Infections
  CMV
  HIV
  C. parvum
  C. neoformans
Other
  Kaposi's sarcoma
  Lymphoma
  Hyperlipidemia
Drugs
  Pentamidine
  Didanosine (DDI, Videx)
  Zalcitabine (DDC, HIVID)
  TMP/SMX

Proctitis
Infections
  HSV
  Neisseria gonorrhea (GC)
  HPV
  Condylomata
  T. pallidum (syphilis)
  Chlamydia trachomatis
  C. parvum
  Microsporidia spp.
  M. avium complex
  CMV

Other
    Kaposi's sarcoma
    Squamous cell cancer of the anorectum

References
1. Hoeprich, pp. 635–637, 642–643. See Bibliography, 1.
2. Kelley, pp. 1645–1651, 1764–1765, 1790–1794,
    1878–1880, 1889–1890. See Bibliography, 2.
3. Schlossberg, pp. 285, 289–292. See Bibliography, 3.
4. Mandell, pp. 1229–1231. See Bibliography, 8.
5. Devita, pp. 356–361, 365–391. See Bibliography, 9.
6. Wormser, pp. 313, 505–527. See Bibliography, 10.
7. Dolin, pp. 767–782. See Bibliography, 15.
8. Hellen HM: Management of Enteric Protozoan Infections,
    pp. 367–377. See Bibliography, 16.

13-F. Central Nervous System Complications

Meningitis
Infections
    Acute HIV infection
    Bacteria, especially *S. pneumoniae, Neisseria meningi-*
        tidis, Haemophilus influenzae
    Listeria monocytogenes
    Salmonella spp.
    Fungal, especially *C. neoformans, H. capsulatum, Candida*
        spp., *Aspergillus* spp., Mucormycoses, *C. immitis*
    Spirochetes, especially *T. pallidum* (syphilis), *B. burgdorferi*
    Mycobacteria, especially *M. tuberculosis, M. avium* com-
        plex, *Mycobacterium kansasii*
Other
    Malignancy, especially lymphoma

Encephalitis
Infections
    HIV
    Herpes simplex virus I (HSV I)
    CMV
    Herpes simplex virus II (HSV II)
    T. gondii
    Papovaviruses [progressive multifocal leukoencephalopa-
        thy (PML)]
    HHV-6

Space-Occupying Lesions
Infections
- *T. gondii*
- *C. neoformans*
- Pyogenic brain abscesses
- *Nocardia asteroides*
- *Salmonella* spp.
- *L. monocytogenes*
- *S. pneumoniae*
- *M. tuberculosis* (tuberculomas)
- *Aspergillus* spp.
- *Streptococcus mitis*
- *Staphylococcus epidermidis*

Other
- Malignancy, especially CNS lymphoma, Kaposi's sarcoma, metastatic cancer
- PML

Myelitis
Infections
- HIV
- CMV
- HSV
- VZV
- *T. pallidum* (syphilis)
- *T. gondii*
- *M. tuberculosis*

Other
- Idiopathic

Infarction, Hemorrhage, Transient Ischemic Attack, Cardiovascular Accident
Infections
- *T. pallidum* vasculitis (syphilis)
- *T. gondii*
- *C. neoformans*
- VZV vasculitis
- *M. tuberculosis*
- *Aspergillus* spp.

Other
- Marantic endocarditis
- Anticardiolipin antibody
- Thrombocytopenia
- Idiopathic

References
1. Hoeprich, pp. 636–641. See Bibliography, 1.
2. Kelley, pp. 1765, 1893. See Bibliography, 2.
3. Schlossberg, pp. 293–295. See Bibliography, 3.
4. Mandell, pp. 1236–1240. See Bibliography, 8.
5. Devita, pp. 331–353. See Bibliography, 9.
6. Wormser, pp. 321–322, 431–473, 621–686. See Bibliography, 10.
7. Sugar, pp. 59–62, 78–82. See Bibliography, 14.
8. Mariuz P, Boster EM, Luft BJ: Toxoplasmosis in HIV-Infected Women, pp. 326–328. See Bibliography, 16.

13-G. Pulmonary Complications

Infections
Pneumonia or pneumonitis
    Bacterial
        S. pneumoniae
        H. influenzae
        S. aureus
        P. aeruginosa
        Escherichia coli
        Legionella spp.
        M. pneumoniae
        C. pneumoniae
        Other gram-negative bacilli
        Nocardia spp., especially *asteroides*
        Rhodococcus equi
    Mycobacteria, especially *M. tuberculosis, M. avium* complex, and *M. kansasii*
    Viral, especially influenza A, B
    Fungal, especially *C. neoformans, H. capsulatum, C. immitis, Aspergillus* spp. (especially *fumigatus*), *Penicillium marneffei, Blastomyces dermatitidis*
    Protozoal, especially *P. carinii, T. gondii*
    Viral, especially CMV, HSV, adenovirus, VZV

Malignancies
    Kaposi's sarcoma
    Lymphoma, especially NHL, Hodgkin's disease
    Bronchogenic carcinoma
    Metastatic carcinoma

Other
  Pulmonary emboli
  Septic pulmonary emboli
  Primary pulmonary hypertension
  Pneumothorax (especially associated with *P. carinii*
        pneumonia)
  Nonspecific interstitial pneumonitis
  Bronchiectasis
  Emphysema
  Lymphocytic interstitial pneumonitis
  Drugs

References

1. Hoeprich, pp. 552, 636–637. See Bibliography, 1.
2. Schlossberg, pp. 297–299. See Bibliography, 3.
3. Goodenberger DH: Pulmonary Aspects, pp. 84–93. See
     Bibliography, 5.
4. Mandell, pp. 1231–1236. See Bibliography, 8.
5. Devita, pp. 260–280, 405–421. See Bibliography, 9.
6. Wormser, pp. 373–388, 389–429. See Bibliography, 10.
7. Sugar, pp. 22–27, 78–80, 89–90. See Bibliography, 14.
8. Feinberg J, Baughman RP: Pulmonary Disease, pp.
     707–721. See Bibliography, 15.

13-H. Dermatologic Complications

Superficial Cutaneous Infections
  Molluscum contagiosum
  HSV I and II
  Cutaneous HPV
  Condyloma
  Candidiasis
  Folliculitis
  VZV
  Bacterial skin infections, especially *S. aureus*
  Dermatophytosis
  Sarcoptes. scabiei (crusted Norwegian scabies)
  Mycobacteria, especially *M. tuberculosis, M. avium* com-
        plex, *Mycobacterium marinum, M. kansasii,
        Mycobacterium hemophilum*
  Cutaneous *P. carinii*
  Impetigo

Systemic Infections with Dermatologic Manifestations
Acute HIV infection
Reiter's syndrome
P. carinii infection
T. pallidum (syphilis)
Bartonella spp.
Bacillary angiomatosis
C. neoformans
H. capsulatum
P. marneffei
M. tuberculosis

Non-Infectious Dermatologic Manifestations
Seborrheic dermatitis
Psoriasis
Pruritus
Atopic dermatitis
Ichythosis-acquired
Porphyria cutanea tarda
Hyperpigmentation
Photodermatitis

Cutaneous Malignancies
Kaposi's sarcoma
B-cell lymphoma
T-cell lymphoma
Invasive squamous cell cancer
Anogenital neoplasia
Basal cell cancer of the skin
Other
Drug reactions, especially pruritus, erythema multiforme,
Stevens-Johnson syndrome, morbilliform rash
Fixed drug eruptions, especially penile ulcers secondary
to Foscarnet
Eosinophilic pustular folliculitis
Toxic epidermal necrolysis
Photosensitivity
Porphyria cutanea tarda
Vitiligo
Thrombocytopenia purpura (TTP)
Bullous pemphigoid
Sicca syndrome
Polyarteritis nodosa
Cutaneous leukocytoclastic vasculitis
Alopecia
Aphthous ulcers

References

1. Hoeprich, pp. 636–637, 646. See Bibliography, 1.
2. Kelley, pp. 1766, 1874, 1888–1892, 1895–1897. See Bibliography, 2.
3. Schlossberg, pp. 296–297. See Bibliography, 3.
4. Pennys NS: Dermatologic Manifestations, pp. 95–100. See Bibliography, 5.
5. Mandell, pp. 1228–1229. See Bibliography, 8.
6. Wormser, pp. 314–317. See Bibliography, 10.
7. Sugar, pp. 34–40. See Bibliography, 14.

13-I. Infections and Complications of Human Immunodeficiency Virus Infection in the 1993 Acquired Immunodeficiency Syndrome Surveillance Definition: Adults and Adolescents*

Candidiasis, esophageal, bronchial, tracheal, pulmonary
Extrapulmonary cryptococcosis
Extrapulmonary coccidioidomycosis
Extrapulmonary or disseminated histoplasmosis
CMV retinitis
HSV bronchitis, pneumonitis, esophagitis, mucocutaneous ulcer of greater than 1-month duration
Isosporiasis or cryptosporidiosis, chronic intestinal of greater than 1-month duration
M. tuberculosis (any site)
Extrapulmonary *M. avium* complex, *M. kansasii*
P. carinii pneumonia
Recurrent bacterial pneumonia, more than two episodes in 1 year
Recurrent *Salmonella* bacteremia
CNS toxoplasmosis
Wasting syndrome secondary to HIV
HIV encephalopathy
Kaposi's sarcoma
Burkitt's lymphoma
Immunoblastic lymphoma
Primary CNS lymphoma
PML

*Adapted from Centers for Disease Control and Prevention, 1993: Revised Classification System for HIV Infection and Expanded Surveillance Case Definition for AIDS Among Adolescents and Adults. MMWR 1992;41(No. RR-17):4–19.

13–J. Indications for the Initiation of Antiretroviral Therapy in the Human Immunodeficiency Virus–Infected Patient

When to initiate therapy		
Clinical category	CD4+ T-cell count and HIV RNA	Recommendation
Symptomatic (AIDS, thrush, unexplained fever)	Any value	Treat.
Asymptomatic	CD4 <500/mm^3 or HIV RNA >20,000 polymerase chain reaction (PCR) or >10,000 branched DNA (bDNA)	Treatment should be encouraged. Strength of recommendation is based on prognosis for disease-free survival and willingness of the patient to accept therapy.
Asymptomatic	CD4 >500/mm^3 and HIV RNA <20,000 (PCR) or <10,000 (bDNA)	Some experts would delay therapy and observe; however, most experts would treat. This would be an aggressive approach.

13-K. Recommended Treatment of Established Human Immunodeficiency Virus Infection*

Column A	Column B
Indinavir	Zidovudine (ZDV) (AZT) + didanosine (DDI)
Nelfinavir	Stavudine (d4T) + DDI
Ritonavir	d4T + lamivudine (3TC)
Ritonavir + saquinavir	ZDV + 3TC
Efavirenz (Sustiva)	Abacavir (Ziagen) + nucleoside reverse transcriptase inhibitor (NRTI)

*Preferred (strong evidence of clinical benefit and sustained suppression of plasma viral load): one highly active protease inhibitor plus two NRTIs (one drug from column A and two from column B). Drugs are listed in random, not priority, order.

Alternative (less well studied; less likely to provide sustained virus suppression): nevirapine or delavirdine + two NRTIs (column B); saquinavir (soft gel cap) + two NRTIs (column B); three NRTIs (still experimental, to include abacavir, with possibly greater toxicity).

Not generally recommended (strong evidence of clinical benefit but initial virus suppression is not sustained in most patients): two NRTIs (column B).

Not recommended (evidence against use, virologically undesirable or overlapping toxicities, or both): all monotherapies, d4T + ZDV, DDC + d4T, DDC + DDI, DDC + 3TC, hard gel capsules of saquinavir (Invirase).

13-L. Characteristics of Nucleoside Reverse Transcriptase Inhibitors

Drug name	Dosing recommendations	Side effects	Laboratory monitoring
Zidovudine (ZDV, AZT, Retrovir)	100 mg; 300-mg capsules; oral suspension, i.v.; 200 mg, p.o. q8h or 300 mg, p.o. q12h. No food or water requirement.	Neutropenia, anemia, headache, fatigue, myalgias, lactic acidosis with hepatic steatosis (rare but potentially fatal).	Complete blood cell count (CBC), liver function tests (LFTs)
Didanosine (DDI, Videx)	25-, 50-, 100-, or 150-mg tablets; 167-mg powdered sachet; ≥60 kg, 200 mg, p.o. q12h; ≤60 kg, 125 mg, p.o. q12h. Take on empty stomach (≥30 min before meal or ≥2 hr after meal).	Pancreatitis, peripheral neuropathy, nausea, diarrhea, abdominal pain, rash, lactic acidosis with hepatic steatosis (rare but potentially fatal).	Lipase ± triglycerides
Zalcitabine [dideoxycytidine (DDC), HIVID]	0.375-mg, 0.75-mg tablets; 0.75 mg, p.o. q8h. Separate DDC and magnesium- or aluminum-containing compounds by ≥1 hr.	Peripheral neuropathy, overlapping toxicity with DDI, d4T causing peripheral neuropathy, stomatitis, anemia, thrombocytopenia, lactic acidosis with hepatic steatosis (rare but potentially fatal).	CBC, lipase

Stavudine (d4T, Zerit)	15-, 20-, 30-, 40-mg tablets ≥60 kg; 40 mg, p.o. q12h ≤60 kg; 30 mg, p.o. q12h.	Overlapping toxicity with DDI, DDC causing peripheral neuropathy, nausea, vomiting, diarrhea, lactic acidosis with hepatic steatosis (rare but potentially fatal).	LFTs, lipase
Lamivudine (3TC, Epivir)	150-mg tablets; 150 mg, p.o. q12h.	Mild rash, headache, diarrhea, lactic acidosis with hepatic steatosis (rare but potentially fatal).	CBC, LFTs
Abacavir (Ziagen)	300-mg tablets; 300 mg, p.o. q12h.	Abacavir hypersensitivity: fever, malaise, rash, fatigue, abdominal pain (do not rechallenge). Headache, nausea, lactic acidosis with hepatic steatosis (rare but potentially fatal).	

13-M. Characteristics of Non-Nucleoside Reverse Transcriptase Inhibitors

Drug name	Dosing recommendations	Side effects	Laboratory monitoring
Nevirapine (NVP, Viramune)	200-mg tablets; 200 mg, p.o. qd × 14 days, then 200 mg, p.o. q12h	Rash, fever, headache, nausea, thrombocytopenia, hepatitis.	CBC, LFTs
Delavirdine (Rescriptor)	100-mg tablets; 400 mg, p.o. q8h on empty stomach; separate administration of antacids, DDI + H₂ blockers by ≥1 hr	Rash, headache, increased LFTs. Contraindicated drugs: rifabutin, rifampin, astemizole, alprazolam, midazolam, cisapride.	LFTs
Efavirenz (Sustiva)	50-, 100-, 200-mg tablets; 600 mg, p.o. qhs	Rash (severe in 5%), insomnia, confusion, dizziness, nightmares, agitation, hallucinations, increased LFTs. Contraindicated drugs: astemizole, triazolam, midazolam, cisapride, ergot alkaloids. Drugs that require monitoring with efavirenz: warfarin, rifampin, rifabutin, clarithromycin, ethinyl, estradiol.	LFTs

13-N. Characteristics of Protease Inhibitors

Drug name	Dosing recommendations	Side effects	Laboratory monitoring
Saquinavir (Fortovase)	200-mg capsules; 120 mg, p.o. t.i.d. Take with high-fat meal. Contraindicated with terfenadine; astemizole can cause risk of arrhythmia. Cisapride, ergot alkaloids, rifampin, rifabutin.	Nausea, diarrhea, abdominal pain, headache, increased LFTs, hyperglycemia, fat redistribution and lipid abnormalities.	CBC; glucose; LFTs; creatine phosphokinase (CPK)
Indinavir (Crixivan)	200-, 400-mg capsules; 800 mg, p.o. q8h 1 hr before or after meals or may take with low-fat snack or meal. Drink 1.5 qt of water per day. If take with DDI, take 2 hr apart. Contraindications: ergot alkaloids, rifampin, astemizole, terfenadine, cisapride, midazolam, triazolam.	Nephrolithiasis, hematuria, headache, nausea, fatigue, dizziness, rash, blurred vision, thrombocytopenia, hyperglycemia, fat redistribution and lipid abnormalities.	Bilirubin (increased indirect bilirubin)
Ritonavir (Norvir)	100-mg capsules, 600 mg/7.5 mL, p.o. solution. Dose escalate: day 1–2 300 mg, p.o. b.i.d.,day 3–5 400 mg, p.o. b.i.d., from day 14 on, on 600 mg, p.o. b.i.d. Take with food.	Nausea, vomiting, diarrhea, paresthesias, circumoral and extremities, altered taste, asthenia, increased LFTs, increased cholesterol, increased triglycerides, increased CPK, uric acid, hyperglycemia,	LFTs, cholesterol, triglycerides, CPK; uric acid

Continued

13-N. Characteristics of Protease Inhibitors (continued)

Drug name	Dosing recommendations	Side effects	Laboratory monitoring
		fat redistribution, and lipid abnormalities. Contraindications: rifampin, rifabutin (decrease dose to one-fourth standard dose), astemizole, cisapride, meperidine, piroxicam, propoxyphene, clozapine, pimozide, alprazolam, diazepam, flurazepam, midazolam, triazolam, clorazepate, zolpidem, ergot alkaloids [dihydroergotamine (DHE) 45, ergotamine (various)], bupropion, amiodarone, flecainide, encainide, quinidine, propafenone].	
Nelfinavir (Viracept)	250-mg tablets; 50-mg/g powder; 1,250 mg, p.o. q12h with food; 750 mg, p.o. q8h with food (or pediatrics 20–30 mg/kg per dose t.i.d. with food).	Mild diarrhea, nausea, hyperglycemia, fat redistribution and lipid abnormalities. Contraindications: terfenadine, astemizole, cisapride (can cause risk of arrhythmias), rifampin, midazolam, triazolam, ergot alkaloids, DHE 45, ergotamine (various forms), decreased levels of ethinyl estradiol and norethindrone, use alternative contraceptive method.	LFTs, CPK

13-O. Drug Interactions between Protease Inhibitors and Other Drugs Requiring Dose Modifications

	Indinavir	Ritonavir	Saquinavir	Nelfinavir
Fluconazole	No dose change	No dose change	No data	No dose change
Ketoconazole and itraconazole	Decrease dose to 600 mg, q8h	Increases ketoconazole greater than threefold; dose adjustment required	Increase saquinavir levels threefold; no dose change	No dose change
Rifabutin	Reduce rifabutin to one-half dose, 150 mg, qd	Consider alternative drug or reduce rifabutin to one-fourth dose, 150 mg q.o.d.	Not recommended with either saquinavir mesylate (Invirase) or saquinavir (Fortovase)	Reduce rifabutin to one-half dose, 150 mg, qd
Rifampin	Contraindicated	Unknown	Not recommended with either Invirase or Fortovase	Contraindicated
Oral contraceptives	Modest increase Ortho-Novum levels; no dose change	Ethinyl estradiol levels decreased; use alternative or additional contraceptive method	No data	Ethinyl estradiol and norethindrone levels decreased; use alternative or additional contraceptive method
Miscellaneous	Grapefruit juice reduces indinavir levels by 26%	Desipramine increased 145%, reduce dose; theophylline levels decreased, increase dose	Grapefruit juice increases saquinavir levels	—

13-P. Drugs That Should Not Be Used with Protease Inhibitors

Drug category	Indinavir	Ritonavir	Saquinavir	Nelfinavir	Alternatives
Analgesics	None	Meperidine, piroxicam, propoxyphene	None	None	Acetylsalicylic acid, oxycodone, acetaminophen
Cardiac	None	Amiodarone, encainide, flecainide, propafenone, quinidine	None	None	Limited experience
Antimycobacterial	Rifampin	Rifabutin, rifampin	Rifampin, rifabutin	Rifampin	For rifabutin: clarithromycin, ethambutol, azithromycin
Ca⁺⁺ channel blocker	None	Bepridil	None	None	Limited experience
Antihistamine	Astemizole, terfenadine	Astemizole, terfenadine	Astemizole, terfenadine	Astemizole, terfenadine	Loratadine, fenofexadine
Gastrointestinal	Cisapride	Cisapride	Cisapride	Cisapride	Limited experience
Antidepressant	None	Bupropion	None	None	Fluoxetine, desipramine

					Limited experience
Neuroleptic	None	Clozapine, pimozide	None	None	
Psychotropic	Midazolam, triazolam	Clorazepate, diazepam, estazolam, flurazepam, midazolam, triazolam, zolpidem, alprazolam	None	Midazolam (Versed), triazolam (Halcion)	Temazepam, lorazepam
Ergot alkaloid (vasoconstrictor)	None	Dihydroergotamine (DHE) 45, ergotamine (various forms)	None	DHE 45, ergotamine (various forms)	None

References

1. Centers for Disease Control and Prevention: The Report of the NIH Panel to Define Principles of Therapy of HIV Infection and Guidelines for the Use of Antiretroviral Agents in HIV-Infected Adults and Adolescents. *MMWR Morb Mortal Wkly Rep* 47:1–32, 1998.
2. Carpenter CJ, Fischl MA, Hammer SM, et al: Antiretroviral Therapy for HIV Infection in 1998: Updated Recommendations of the International AIDS Society—U S A Panel. *JAMA* 280:78–86, 1998.
3. Flexner C: HIV-Protease Inhibitors. *N Engl J Med* 338:1281–1292, 1998.
4. See Bibliography, 1.
5. See Bibliography, 5.
6. See Bibliography, 6.
7. See Bibliography, 10.
8. Devita: Pharmacology of Antiretroviral Agents, pp. 479–493. See Bibliography, 9.
9. Inouye RT, Hammer SM: Initiation of Therapy, pp. 248–246. See Bibliography, 15
10. See Bibliography, 17.
11. Wormser, pp. 296–302. See Bibliography, 10.
12. Wormser, pp. 717–732. See Bibliography, 10.

Bibliography

1. Hoeprich PD, Jordan CM, Ronald AR: *Infectious Diseases: A Treatise of Infectious Processes*, 5/e. Philadelphia: JB Lippincott Co, 1994.
2. Kelley WN. *Textbook of Internal Medicine*, 3/e. Philadelphia: Lippincott–Raven, 1997.
3. Schlossberg D, Shulman JA: *Differential Diagnosis of Infectious Diseases*, 1/e. Philadelphia: Williams & Wilkins, 1996.
4. Carey CF, Lee HH, Woeltje KF (eds): *The Washington Manual of Infectious Diseases*, 1/e. Philadelphia: Lippincott–Raven, 1998.
5. Powderly WG (ed): *Manual of HIV Therapeutics*. Philadelphia: Lippincott–Raven, 1997.
6. Gilbert DN, Moellering RC, Sande MA: *The Sanford Guide to Antimicrobial Therapy* 1999, 29/e. Hyde Park, VT: Antimicrobial Therapy, 1998.
7. Reese RE, Betts RF: *A Practical Approach to Infectious Diseases*, 4/e. New York: Little, Brown and Company, 1996.

8. Mandell GL, Bennett JE, Dolin R: *Principles and Practices of Infectious Diseases*, 4/e. New York: Churchill Livingstone, 1995.

9. Devita VT, et al: *AIDS: Etiology, Diagnosis, Treatment and Prevention*, 4/e. Philadelphia: Lippincott–Raven, 1997.

10. Wormser GP (ed): *AIDS and Other Manifestations of HIV Infection*, 3/e. Philadelphia: Lippincott–Raven, 1998.

11. Bartlett JG: *Pocket Book of Infectious Disease Therapy*. Philadelphia: Williams & Wilkins, 1997.

12. Mandell LA, Niederman MS (eds): *Infectious Disease Clinics of North America: Lower Respiratory Tract Infections*. Philadelphia: Williams & Wilkins, 1998.

13. Gold JWM, Telzak EE, White DA (eds): *The Medical Clinics of North America: Management of the HIV-Infected Patient, Part II. Infections and Malignancies Associated with HIV Infection*. Philadelphia: WB Saunders, 1997.

14. Sugar AM, Lyman CA: *A Practical Guide to Medically Important Fungi and the Diseases They Cause*. Philadelphia: Lippincott–Raven, 1997.

15. Dolin R, Massur H, Saag MS: *AIDS Therapy*. Philadelphia: Churchill Livingstone, 1999.

16. Cotton D, Watts DH: *The Medical Management of AIDS in Women*. New York: Wiley–Liss, 1997.

17. Bartlett JG: *1999 Medical Management of HIV Infection*. Baltimore: Johns Hopkins University, Department of Infectious Diseases, 1999.

INDEX